THE

DASH
DIET
Mediterranean
Solution

Also by Marla Heller

The DASH Diet Younger You

The Everyday DASH Diet Cookbook

The DASH Diet Weight Loss Solution

The DASH Diet Action Plan

THE
DASH
DIET
Mediterranean
Solution

THE BEST EATING PLAN
TO **CONTROL YOUR WEIGHT**
AND **IMPROVE YOUR HEALTH**
FOR LIFE

Marla Heller, MS, RD

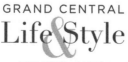

GRAND CENTRAL
Life & Style
NEW YORK · BOSTON

Grand Central Life & Style
Hachette Book Group
1290 Avenue of the Americas, New York, NY 10104
grandcentrallifeandstyle.com
twitter.com/grandcentralpub

First Edition: December 2018

Grand Central Life & Style is an imprint of Grand Central Publishing. The Grand Central Life & Style name and logo are trademarks of Hachette Book Group, Inc.

The publisher is not responsible for websites (or their content) that are not owned by the publisher.

The Hachette Speakers Bureau provides a wide range of authors for speaking events. To find out more, go to www.hachettespeakersbureau.com or call (866) 376-6591.

Library of Congress Control Number: 2018952141

ISBNs: 978-1-5387-1525-3 (hardcover), 978-1-5387-1524-6 (ebook)

Printed in the United States of America

LSC-H

10 9 8 7 6 5 4 3 2 1

*To my husband, Richard, who makes
our life together so much fun.*

CONTENTS

PART 1

CHAPTER 1:   The Best of the Best   3

CHAPTER 2:   Getting to the Heart of the Matter   19

CHAPTER 3:   The New Philosophy for Reaching and
             Maintaining a Healthy Weight for
             the Rest of Your Life!   37

CHAPTER 4:   Surprising Benefits of the Med-DASH Plan   45

CHAPTER 5:   Want Different Results? Do Things
             Differently!   63

CHAPTER 6:   The Big Three   77

CHAPTER 7:   Real Food, Real Easy   89

CHAPTER 8:   The Super-Simple Overview:
             Med-DASH Rules   101

PART 2

CHAPTER 9:   Optional Jump-Start and Relearning
             How to Eat   109

CHAPTER 10: The Full Med-DASH Eating Plan   127

CHAPTER 11: On Autopilot: Make It Easy and Simple!   153

CHAPTER 12: Problems No More!   169

CHAPTER 13: Recipes: Make It Delicious!   177

CHAPTER 14: Your Best Health: The Med-DASH
             Impact   227

APPENDIX A. Beef   233

APPENDIX B. Pork   235

APPENDIX C. Poultry   237

APPENDIX D. Seafood Composition   239

APPENDIX E. Sources of Omega-3 Fats   241

APPENDIX F. Good Sources of Calcium, Potassium,
             and Magnesium   243

Notes   245
Acknowledgments   251
Index   253
About the Author   263

PART 1

CHAPTER 1

The Best of the Best

The DASH diet (based on the research, Dietary Approaches to Stop Hypertension) and the Mediterranean diet have both been acclaimed as the best of the best in the world. Both became famous for their amazing impact on heart health. Both help reduce inflammation and are associated with lower rates of heart attacks, strokes, heart failure, certain types of cancer, and a reduced risk of developing type 2 diabetes. Following these eating patterns has been shown to help preserve brain health. And as you will learn here, together they comprise a plan that is sustainable, so that it will become your life-long healthy eating style while helping you reach and maintain a healthy weight.

There is so much confusion about diets. How can we know if we have a good one, when it seems like every time we turn around, there is a new hot diet in the news? What does it mean to say that one or two diets are the best? Are they really better than any other diet, or might the nutrition gurus say something entirely different next year? And beyond the hype, how can we, ourselves, judge if a diet is really good? We've seen this happen over and over. A diet is super popular, and then after a few years you never hear about that miracle diet again.

Would it reassure you to know that there are only two diets that have stood the test of time? And that they are completely compatible, complementary, and even better together? Why not choose the best of the best? This is the moment to change your life.

The DASH diet and the Mediterranean diet are the plans that endure. Year after year. They have stood atop the best diet rankings every year that the panel of experts from *U.S. News & World Report* has rated all the popular and also-ran diets. The DASH diet is extra rich in fruits and vegetables, low-fat dairy, and nuts, and includes mostly whole grains, lean meats, fish, and poultry, and moderate amounts of heart-healthy fats. The Mediterranean diet is also based on all those foods, along with an emphasis on seafood, olive oil, beans, herbs, and spices, and the optional inclusion of red wine. When you combine DASH with the Mediterranean diet, you truly have the best of the best. Not a fad. The *only* diets that have stood up under scrutiny. Because they work and have been proven to work in multiple, multiple studies. No diets have been this researched. No other diets have this kind of medical pedigree. Even better together, they help people get healthier and support reaching and maintaining a healthy weight. Easily. Deliciously.

Don't be fooled!

A diet is a food pattern. An eating style. It doesn't just refer to a weight-loss plan. The DASH eating pattern can be for everyone, as can the Mediterranean.

For any diet or eating pattern to be worth your time and effort, it should be something you can live with for the long run, and it should make you healthier. No plan should be so restrictive or difficult that it leads to feeling bad about yourself or induces guilt if you don't follow it perfectly. No plan should ruin your health. (Even if you only follow it for a short while.) It's only a worthy plan if it makes you feel great and lets you truly enjoy eating. It should help you set the stage for continued success, not set you up for failure.

The Mediterranean DASH diet—"Med-DASH"—plan is all of that. It is a delicious, enjoyable, beautiful way of eating, and it just happens to make you healthier. There are no other plans in the world with the same proven health benefits or that address each of our epidemic chronic health issues. This plan makes it easy to manage weight and reduces risk for heart disease, hypertension, fatty liver disease,[1] and diabetes. If your goal is to reach or sustain a healthy weight, the Med-DASH plan is so satisfying that you will find it's easy to stay on track with your goals. You will relearn how to eat, how to set the stage for success even in a busy life, how to enjoy restaurant meals, and how to continue to follow this plan because it makes you feel better and you love eating this way. You will discover positive changes in your body and how it operates. This plan has been proven to lower cholesterol and blood sugar. Your waistline will shrink, which is a huge clue that your body is better able to metabolize carbohydrates instead of storing extra glucose in your abdominal (visceral) fat and your liver. Belly fat is the symptom, but diabetes, high blood pressure, clogged arteries, and fatty liver disease are the consequences.

Forget struggling, forget "cheating," forget counting calories, forget lists of allowed and forbidden foods, forget the battle to follow one more diet that gives guidance that completely conflicts with sound science regarding what your body does and doesn't need to get healthy. Forget those feelings of failure that you had when you found that the latest fad diet was impossible to stick with. This plan has a positive focus, with negativity banished from dieting.

You are going to love, love, love this plan. The Mediterranean

DASH diet is a fresh way of eating that relies on solid nutrition science to propel you to reach your goals. Scientifically proven and translated into fabulous meals, the Med-DASH plan provides all the strategies you need to facilitate your entry into the delicious new world of healthy eating.

What is the promise of the Med-DASH program? Heart health is what garnered all the attention for the DASH diet and the Mediterranean diet. Lower blood pressure. Lower cholesterol. Reduced rates of heart attack, stroke, and heart failure. And there is so much more. Research shows that DASH is associated with improved brain health and reduced systemic inflammation, along with lower risk for type 2 diabetes, some types of cancers, and fatty liver disease. This is the way healthy people have been eating for generations. Before all the processed foods and easy access to junk food. Back when food was slow and delicious.

Does this seem like a miracle? It may be, but it is based on the real-life results observed by studying how the healthiest people have eaten over the years. Do they eat more vegetables? Check! More fruits? Check! Healthy, protein-rich foods? Check! Add to that the fats that are beneficial for your heart, particularly from olive oil, avocados, nuts, and seafood. The Mediterranean people usually complement their meals with red wine—which is completely optional, but you can do that on this program if you'd like. All these habits combine to make a complete program or eating style that you will love and appreciate for your health, your well-being, and your gastronomic pleasure.

I have heard that this eating pattern just seems like common sense. Yes, it is. But unfortunately, common-sense eating is very uncommon. It isn't our habit. We didn't get our epidemics of heart disease, diabetes, and obesity by following common-sense principles regarding the majority of our decisions about how to eat. Sadly, too many people have missed out on the best, flexible eating plans because up until now, no one made them into a real-life, practical, and delicious lifestyle program. People have avoided even trying either the DASH diet or the Mediterranean diet, perhaps because they thought the plans might be too difficult, confusing, or not enjoyable enough.

The epidemics of chronic disease are the result of our having destroyed our bodies with low-level inflammation that is mostly the result of unhealthy eating. This inflammation is the root cause of plaque buildup in the arteries. Inflammation causes the body to store excess carbs as belly fat (also called visceral fat) and leads to fatty liver disease, both of which are associated with the development of type 2 diabetes. Inflammation is considered to be a factor in initiating some cancers, including some types of breast cancer and colorectal cancer. Poor diet and unhealthy weight are at the root of this inflammation. We need to reexamine how we eat and find out how to make it easy to follow a realistic, healthy eating plan. We need a sane plan that is time-proven, with self-evident health benefits.

You are going to wipe out your memory of all the bad diet advice from the past. Too many diets encourage eating lots of processed starchy foods, cutting way down on fats, and eating lower amounts of protein-rich foods. This was a recipe for making meals that were less satisfying, leading to overeating and weight struggles at levels never before seen in the U.S. Between 1979 and 2014, the U.S. adult obesity rate increased from 15 percent to nearly 38 percent, with the fastest increase coming after 1988.[2] But the weight problem is only a symptom of impending chronic diseases. Following those old high-carb guidelines, for many people, wore out the body's ability to produce insulin, resulting in type 2 diabetes or prediabetes. And in fact, the number of adult Americans diagnosed with diabetes increased from 5 million to 23 million between 1979 and 2014. And we know that the real number is twice as high, since about half of actual cases are undiagnosed. So forget loading up on carbs or skimping on fats or protein. That advice needs to be erased from your memory banks. Banished!

While we're at it, let's wipe our memories of all the fad diets from the last two decades. Why were we so eager to jump on the bandwagon for fad diets that we knew weren't healthy and that conflicted with the standard USDA recommendations from the food guidelines? Why did we think we could get results that we were happy with on programs that were so clearly unsustainable? To some degree, the issue is that we simply didn't believe the national food guidelines could be a workable model for how we should eat. People were skeptical because it seemed that the USDA was too much in the pockets of lobbyists for the processed food industry and grain farmers. Yes, the feds were much too slow to warn people about excessive sugar and refined grain products in our diets. They were too slow to strongly embrace vegetarian diets and organic foods. When dietary guidelines were developed, the DASH and Mediterranean diets only showed up buried in the fine print or footnotes of very dense reports. The oversimplified and vague nutrition guidance was unhelpful. Fad diets proliferated in the absence of beneficial national nutrition guidelines.

Neither the DASH diet nor the Mediterranean diet was brought to you by any lobbyist. Nor were they promoted by advertising or highly paid publicity agents. These two plans, DASH and Med, were created by looking at what the healthiest people eat and have eaten over long periods of time. But sadly, these scientific breakthroughs were just languishing, waiting for someone to turn them into real-life solutions, with, perhaps, a little of the glamour of the fad diets.

Many of the fad diets have been focused on the "don't eat" principle. Don't eat gluten. Don't eat meat. Don't eat foods that ever had a face. Don't eat animal foods at all. Don't eat white foods. Don't eat nightshade foods. Surprise! We are not going there. We will focus on the "let's eat" principle—what you *should* include. A positive focus that prioritizes delicious, vibrant, beautiful eating.

When I decided to become a dietitian, my motivation was to show people how to eat in a healthy way and make it enjoyable.

I was struck by how many of my coworkers were having heart attacks at relatively young ages, but still would not change anything in their eating or activity habits to avoid future events. They felt they would rather continue to eat the foods they loved than change to a "boring, unappealing" healthy diet. They chose not to lose weight or protect their hearts. Unfortunately, they died of massive heart attacks, much too young. That is why I believe it is imperative that we change our perceptions about the false choice between being healthy and enjoying food. My mission is to show you that healthy eating can be fabulous! Because if you don't enjoy it, you won't follow the plan, and that does no one any good.

And lest you think heart disease is something only men have to worry about, heart disease is the number one killer of women, too. And over two-thirds of women who have a heart attack will never fully recover.[3,4] Heart disease kills more people than all types of cancer combined. (More on this later.)

Let's move on to a plan that will promote heart health and be a pleasure to follow. It must deliver on this seemingly impossible promise, or why bother? This has been the mission of my career and my mission in writing this book. And I am thrilled to be able to share this secret with you.

It's Not a Secret Anymore!

The DASH diet and the Mediterranean diet are the two most researched diets in history. They weren't discovered as a result of some happy accident in a science lab. Rather, their discoveries were based on observations of how regular people live and eat in various parts of the world, and how that affects their health. It has been well-known that people in certain regions live longer and are healthy for their entire lives. What has been discovered about the secrets for a healthy life?

In the Mediterranean region, especially Sardinia in Italy and

Crete and Corfu in Greece, people continue to follow a traditional eating pattern, one that is rich in plant foods, along with cheese and yogurts, seafood, and limited amounts of meat. Their diets also include lots of salad greens, herbs, and spices. And of course, wine and coffee are also stalwarts of the daily lives of people in the Mediterranean region. People in these regions are also usually physically active and very socially connected. Many of them live to be over ninety or even one hundred, and are still in good health.

Another Mediterranean country with lower rates of heart problems is France. They eat lots of cheese, meat, and white bread, yet they do not suffer from high rates of heart disease. This is described as the French Paradox. Of course, they eat moderate portions and are famous for their green salads (*salades vertes*) with every meal. They are also likely to have fruit for dessert and snacks. They include vegetables with their meals, have regular consumption of coffee and wine, and walk everywhere. When you are on the streets of Paris, you are struck by all the flat bellies. So different from the plump bellies we see on most Americans, which are not just a size issue, but are indicators of metabolic illness.

Of course, not all Americans have these problems. We can find clusters of super-healthy people who live among us, but with a few different lifestyle choices. In the United States, it was observed that there was a population that seemed to be blessed with longevity and health. In the region of Loma Linda, California, there were many people living to be over one hundred years old in good physical health. This area is home to many Seventh-Day Adventists, who are primarily vegetarian. Like traditional Italians and Greeks, they are physically active and socially connected. What is so special about these people's habits that seems to protect them from the ailments that befall most Americans? What has allowed them to have lower blood pressure and lower rates of heart disease? They don't live in a bubble. They get their foods from the same food supply as the rest of Americans and are subject to the same stresses of everyday life. But, as noted, they are primarily vegetarian. They are physically active throughout their day, not just through exercise, but with their chores around the house, walking places, hiking, enjoying nature.

The DASH diet is a specific eating pattern, rich in plant-based foods, which was originally designed to lower blood pressure without medication. It was, additionally, designed to be the healthiest possible diet that would be acceptable to the eating style of the average American. It well-known that traditional vegetarians living in the United States live longer and have fewer chronic diseases than the average American. A vegetarian diet formed the basis of the DASH diet. However, researchers knew that most Americans wouldn't want to follow such a strict plan, so DASH also incorporates meats, poultry, and fish. It is extra rich in fruits and vegetables, and includes dairy, beans, nuts and seeds, mostly whole grains, and heart-healthy fats.

The DASH diet delivers the vegetarian benefits, but without making you give up some favorite foods (although it fully supports a wholly vegetarian eating plan, if that's what you want).

The Mediterranean and the DASH diet plans are so similar that it seems perfect to put them together. Who wouldn't want the promise of longer, healthier life? Who wouldn't want the promise of being able to reduce or eliminate dependency on medications? But of course, we want the plan to be something we can actually follow in a real life, with all of its time challenges, and it should accommodate our own personal tastes and food preferences. We want a plant-based diet, with some flexibility, and we are completely willing to incorporate olive oil to make our meals more satisfying.

Our two mash-up plans:

1. The DASH diet—Developed in research, to provide benefits that were observed from plant-focused and vegetarian diets and designed to be America's healthiest diet.

2. The Mediterranean diet—Discovered via observation of the habits of some of the world's healthiest and longest-lived people.

Each is plant-focused and includes beans, nuts, and seeds; dairy; olive oil and other heart-healthy fats; as well as seafood and moderate amounts of meats for those who choose to include them. Both are associated with lower risks for cardiovascular disease and type 2 diabetes.

The first publication of DASH research was in 1997. It was immediately seen as a breakthrough program for an epidemic health problem. DASH was even incorporated into the U.S. treatment guidelines for hypertension, mandated for all physicians.[5] Now it is over twenty years later, and the *Journal of the American Medical Association* recently published an editorial bemoaning the fact that DASH has never received widespread use. Many physicians, in spite of knowing the DASH diet's strong health benefits, do not often prescribe it because they think it is too hard to follow. Based on the strong research evidence, DASH has been a consistent part of U.S. national treatment guidelines and U.S. dietary recommendations since the original publication of the diet's supporting research.[6] I first heard about the DASH diet from my advisor for my master's degree thesis, Shiriki Kumanyika, PhD, MPH, RD. As one of the foremost researchers on the relationship between diet and blood pressure, she was involved in the creation of the DASH eating pattern. But even before the first research about the DASH diet was published, it had been my mission to make it easy to follow and practical for real lives; a plan that can become a life-long eating style. Although over six hundred thousand of my books have been sold, DASH is still an unexplored topic for too many people. It is my belief that DASH could and should be the foundation for how we eat in this country—not as a weight-loss tool or a program to regulate chronic illnesses we already have, but as the foundation for sensible eating for every man, woman, and child. This is a philosophy about food that can optimize health for everyone—why wait until you have a problem that needs to be solved?

The health benefits seem almost miraculous. DASH controls high blood pressure as well as the first-line medications. Let that sink in. *As well as the first-line medications!* The 2017 blood pressure treatment guidelines for stage 1 hypertension recommend the DASH diet, along with the Mediterranean diet, as part of the lifestyle strategies for controlling the "silent killer." DASH also helps lower cholesterol and is associated with reduced risk of strokes, heart attacks, heart failure, some kinds of cancer, type 2 diabetes, and kidney stones. And though not originally designed as a weight-loss plan, DASH easily adapts, and helps people reach and maintain a healthy weight. It provides more satisfying meals and snacks, which make it easy to manage hunger and avoid overeating. Who would not want all these benefits in one package?

The Mediterranean diet has also been shown to be directly associated with many health benefits. Heart health and longevity were the first observed benefits. New studies have suggested that the Mediterranean diet may help stave off the deterioration of cognitive function on aging, and perhaps even Alzheimer's disease. It may help relieve depression and reduce the risk for colon cancer.

Let's learn a little more...

The DASH Diet

In the mid-1990s, the DASH diet (Dietary Approaches to Stop Hypertension)[7] was conceived as a way to help lower blood pressure through a healthy diet rather than with medication. The researchers had been investigating the effect of diet on blood pressure for some time. Now it was time to put this knowledge into action.

The researchers had also noted that diets rich in calcium and potassium and to a lesser extent, magnesium, were beneficial for lowering blood pressure. It seemed logical to evaluate whether taking supplements of these nutrients would lower blood pressure. Several studies were conducted, but unfortunately, most showed little or no benefit from calcium, potassium, or magnesium supplementation, so the focus returned to diet.

As we have noted, it was observed that, in general, vegetarians living in the United States had lower blood pressure and lower rates of heart disease mortality than people eating a more traditional Western diet. But few Americans would be willing to give up meat even if it meant reducing the risk of a heart attack. Being frustrated with the failure of supplements to provide an easy solution for high blood pressure, the researchers decided to create a diet that was rich in the foods containing those nutrients. The diet was replete with plant foods, including fruits, vegetables, beans, nuts, seeds, mostly whole grains, and heart-healthy oils. Reduced-fat dairy was an essential part of the diet, along with limited amounts of lean meats and poultry, and fish. It was based on the knowledge learned about vegetarian diets.

The first research on the DASH diet was published in 1997. The goal of that study was to evaluate the effect of the diet pattern on blood pressure, and it did so very effectively. The DASH diet lowered blood pressure as well as the first-line blood pressure medications, and in only fourteen days. Amazingly, the blood pressure breakthrough occurred even though the researchers did not allow the participants to lose weight. It incorporated lots of carbs, specifically to avoid weight loss, because if the participants had also lost weight, the researchers would not have known whether the weight loss or the eating pattern was the beneficial aspect. According to *New England Journal of Medicine*: "DASH was particularly effective for those with hypertension (SBP and DBP change: –10.7 and –4.7 mm Hg, respectively)."[8]

In the late 1980s and 1990s most heart specialists were recommending replacing saturated fats (SFA) with what were then called complex carbohydrates. Later research (Omni-Heart) was conducted to evaluate if DASH diet blood pressure results would be better if, instead of replacing SFA with carbs (particularly refined carbs), SFA were replaced with monounsaturated fats (MUFA) or protein. And indeed, they did see better results.[9,10] Both approaches lowered total cholesterol, but MUFA did not increase triglycerides (TG) or lower "good" cholesterol (HDL). Keeping HDL higher and TG lower is very beneficial for heart health and is an important sign that you are successfully managing or lowering your risk for metabolic syndrome. A special benefit was that appetite seemed to be much easier to control.

Instead of needing medication that had some very undesirable side effects, the participants could have very positive "side benefits." Wouldn't you like to keep your blood pressure under control with food rather than with medication? Had you ever heard about the DASH diet before you picked up this book? Most people have not.

So why hasn't DASH adoption been more widespread? Why hasn't it broken out? Most of the educational materials, including those from the National Heart, Lung, and Blood Institute (NHLBI), made DASH seem difficult to follow. (When I first used the NHLBI literature, I found my patients' eyes glazed over.) Based on the complicated information provided in that literature, many doctors felt that it would be too difficult for patients to follow, so they don't even bother to recommend it. *What a shame!* I thought. *This eating pattern is too important to just be a research curiosity.* I wrote my first book on DASH to show people how easy it could be to adopt as a life-long pattern. And it worked. People found that they could stick with it and that their health improved dramatically. So let's continue to follow up on the newest improvements on DASH and incorporate the key Mediterranean diet foods to make this the best plan ever! And the best-tasting!

The Mediterranean Diet

It has been long known that people who live in the Mediterranean region have lower rates of heart disease than people eating a typical Western diet. Since it is a totally delicious way of eating, it can be a great model of how to eat. It would be helpful to learn what the key health factors are and how it works. You can probably guess that it isn't the pasta and white bread that make it effective. After World War II, one of the foremost nutrition scientists in the world, Ancel Keys, organized a consortium of researchers in several countries to investigate how diet impacted health. During World War II, Dr. Keys had become especially famous for designing military K-rations, and for determining how to nutritionally restore the starving people who would soon be liberated from concentration camps. Under the bleachers at the football stadium of the University of Minnesota, Dr. Keys designed a program to begin successfully refeeding starving people, using volunteers from the ranks of conscientious objectors as his subjects. After the war, Dr. Keys was ready to spearhead pursuing foundational nutrition research to learn how the eating patterns in various countries affected heart health. Thus began the Seven Countries Study.

Some of the key findings of the study were learning more details about the types of foods included in a traditional Mediterranean diet, the foods that influenced the risk for heart attacks and other types of heart disease. Important features were that people ate lots of fruits and vegetables, including lots of different types of salad greens, and consumed lots of olive oil. They ate small amounts of meat but enjoyed seafood more frequently. Dr. Keys noticed that the only negative feature about the Mediterranean eating style was that Italy had the highest rate of obesity in Europe, even in postwar Europe when most people did not have enough to eat. Unlike with a more traditional eating style, the Italians tended to have excessive consumption of refined grain foods, such as bread and pasta, which were plentiful and inexpensive. Throughout the region, people complained that they did not get enough meat or poultry and would have loved to have it be more available and more affordable.

Now we know that we can take the best of the Mediterranean plan (without the excessive refined foods that are not traditional and with a little more of the protein-rich foods) to get all the heart-health benefits without weight gain. A recent study showed that the heart-health benefits of the Mediterranean diet are equally good with the inclusion of more lean meats.[11]

Reaping the Benefits

The DASH diet and the Mediterranean diet are the two of the most healthful diets and the ones that have been most researched to learn all the amazing benefits. They both offer the promise of longer, healthier life. Combining them into a new healthy eating style, along with being physically active, makes a true fountain of youth. With the Med-DASH plan, it's not about the bread and pasta. Instead we will focus on the foods key to the Mediterranean diet: colorful vegetables, fruit, fish, nuts and beans, olive oil, and lots of herbs and spices.

There are so many misunderstandings about what the Mediterranean diet incorporates. First, drop your image of a Mediterranean diet as being heaping plates of pasta with lots of bread. Sorry, but that's not it. The real soul of the heart-healthy Med diet pattern is the plant-based foods, like a variety of salad greens, high-fiber beans, and other vegetables, such as in our recipes for Greek Black-Eyed Pea Salad (page 185), Moroccan Chickpea and Green Bean Salad with Ras el Hanout (page 186), Tabil-Spiced Pork Tenderloin with White Beans and Harissa (page 207), or Sautéed Chicken with Tomatoes over Haricots Verts (page 200), followed by a dessert of fresh fruit such as sliced peaches or pears. Add to that plenty of olive oil (it's not a low-fat diet!), seafood such as Spanish-Style Pan-Roasted Cod (page 198), and fermented dairy, including Greek yogurt. And, of course, this is high-flavor eating, rich in herbs and spices. There is a huge variety of fabulous foods, since the Mediterranean region includes Greece, France, Italy, and Spain in Europe, as well as North Africa and the countries around the Eastern Mediterranean. Our recipe collection will help you take some interesting culinary journeys through this food world.

You will love following this delicious eating pattern, which absolutely helps make it so easy to adopt this plan for a lifetime. It is naturally satisfying and health promoting, and miles away from the old dietary guidelines that led to the epidemics of overweight and obesity, heart disease, and type 2 diabetes. This is the way of eating you should be following for the rest of your life!

In this book, I will share with you the best wisdom from my bestselling DASH diet books, along with brand-new guidelines, ideas, and recipes that incorporate the Mediterranean diet and lifestyle. If you are coming to this book because your doctor told you that you need to deal with your blood pressure, cholesterol, or other chronic diseases, welcome. I hope to make your transition into a new way of eating easy, delicious, and exciting. If you are here because you are looking for ways to be healthier, welcome to you, too! The tools and strategies in this book have been working for decades (even centuries!) to help people live happy, healthy, long lives. Together we will explore those habits and create new guidelines for your everyday life. No matter what brought you here, I'm so glad you've come. Let's begin!

CHAPTER 2

Getting to the Heart of the Matter

Heart disease is epidemic in the United States and around the world. It might seem self-evident, but your lifestyle habits have a huge impact on your health, especially heart health. You may think you can wait until later, maybe until you get into late middle age, to live more healthfully. While adopting good habits at any point in your life can be beneficial, why not start right now to keep yourself as young as possible for as long as you can? Research that has followed people for very long periods time, tracking their health, diets, and activity levels, has shown that following the DASH or the Mediterranean diet is associated with lower risks for heart attacks, stroke, and heart failure. We know that the DASH diet specifically improves blood pressure, and that it is associated with lower "bad" (LDL) cholesterol and better "good" (HDL) cholesterol. Follow-up DASH research showed that replacing refined carbs with monounsaturated fats (MUFA) or extra protein improved blood pressure and HDL, while lowering triglycerides.[1] This is a particularly beneficial improvement on the DASH diet, and it has been fully implemented in this Med-DASH diet plan.

Let's learn a little bit about heart disease. Your arteries can take decades to get to the point of being so blocked that they can start to limit blood flow to parts of your heart muscle and other areas of your body. Long before you are close to having a major blockage and a potential heart attack, you may notice you feel very tired and are easily fatigued. You may think you are just getting older and need to slow down, but in reality, it may be time to go see a cardiologist for a battery of tests. He or she will likely do an EKG, which may lead to a stress test and possibly a nuclear stress test. While we would prefer not to need either, it's much better to discover you have a blockage via a test, rather than finding out during a heart attack. That heart attack will leave part of your heart muscle with dead tissue. You may never be the same; the majority of women who have heart attacks will never fully recover to their level of health before the attack. The best prevention strategy is to change your habits now. I will make this easy, and at the same time provide you with guidance on how to enjoy delicious food using this eating pattern.

When I worked at a Navy hospital, I was shocked to hear some of the sailors say they were starting to slow down because they were in their late thirties or early forties and ready to retire from their military career. I was in my fifties at the time, and I was much more energetic and fit than these young men. I saw retirees and their spouses who were younger than me but looked twenty years older. Using canes, with limited mobility, these men and women were much too old before their time. But on the positive side, I also saw a retired couple who were in their late nineties, very physically fit and full of life, always planning their next trips. They stopped by once a year to be sure that they were doing the best they could to stay young. And they were not alone. I saw many people who were in their seventies, eighties, and nineties and doing their best to stay active. One of our friends is a ninety-three-year-old man with an encyclopedic knowledge of baseball and a ready collection of jokes. In addition to joining our coffee group every morning for his social well-being, every day he walks in his community pool for an hour. He says that if he didn't do that, he wouldn't be able to walk at all. He has decided to stay young. Another friend is an eighty-seven-year-old former Marine who golfs eighteen holes (without a cart!) three to five times per week, early in the morning before he joins the group at coffee. Being active, social, and fit is a choice, and helps give pleasure to life. These experiences are seared into my brain and have reinforced my actions to extend my own health and longevity. We need to take another look at our expectations and decide to stay young and healthy for our entire lives. We can do it. Even if heart disease or diabetes runs in your family, you can change what happens to you. Having a genetic disposition toward heart disease is like having a bare piece of land. You can plant seeds and tend the garden, or you can let it go to weeds. It's up to you. Following the Med-DASH diet will prevent those heart disease "weeds" and reduce your risk for developing cardiovascular problems by letting your good health and well-being grow.

The Big Picture

One of the reasons the DASH-Med plan is so important is the very high prevalence of diseases that can be managed by it. The most recent estimates[2] of the impact of these lifestyle-related diseases in the United States are:

- Cardiovascular disease: 93 million people, or about 37 percent of the U.S. adult population, at a cost of about $330 billion per year. Cardiovascular disease is the number one cause of death in the United States, higher than all types of cancer combined, for men *and* for women.

- Hypertension: 86 million Americans, with an annual health-care cost of $53 billion.
- Type 2 diabetes: about 30 million people, including those who are undiagnosed, plus 82 million people with prediabetes. The annual cost is about $245 billion.
- Metabolic syndrome: almost 35 percent of adult Americans.[3]

While these are statistics, the consequences are far more devastating: heart attack, stroke, kidney failure, amputations, blindness, intolerable nerve pain. You don't want to go down this road. Your life will never be the same. Let's get out in front of this!

Cardiovascular Disease

When we consider our personal risk for heart disease, we have factors that we can and cannot change, as shown in table 1.

Heart Disease Risk Factors	
Risks we cannot change	*Risks we can change or manage*
Getting older	Diet
Family history	Exercise
Biologically male	Use of tobacco
Chronic kidney disease	Weight
Sleep apnea*	Cholesterol and triglycerides
Lower socioeconomic status	Blood pressure
	Diabetes

* The newest AHA guidelines note that treating sleep apnea does not reduce the risk of heart disease.

Table 1

The major concerns around cardiovascular disease include heart attacks, peripheral artery disease (PAD), strokes, and heart failure. The important measures we use to judge whether we are doing the right things to manage heart health include monitoring blood pressure, cholesterol, triglycerides, pulse rate, etc. Having high blood pressure, also called hypertension, makes you much more likely to have a stroke or heart failure (and kidney failure). Hypertension is a particularly debilitating disease. If your heart becomes less efficient, it may end up having a hard time pushing your blood through your circulatory system. Then fluid starts building up in your lungs, making it difficult to breathe. This disease, if not well managed, typically results in frequent hospitalizations. Heart failure will make you feel much older and can severely limit your activities and even lead to premature death.

These conditions are often called silent killers because if you don't have regular physical exams, you will probably not be aware of having elevated blood pressure, cholesterol, and/or triglycerides until you have an event like a stroke or a heart attack. Just because you feel all right does not mean you can or should avoid regular checkups with your doctor. You would much rather prevent a problem than have to deal with very severe consequences.

Know Your Numbers!

A key objective of this book is to help you keep your heart healthy. The primary problems that we are trying to manage or avoid are atherosclerosis, high blood pressure, and metabolic syndrome. The main numbers you need to know include your total cholesterol, LDL cholesterol (the bad type), HDL cholesterol (the good type since it helps to clean up arteries), and triglyceride, all of which are collectively known as blood lipids. Blood glucose and blood pressure are the other important numbers to know.

Your physician will set targets for your blood lipids depending on your personal medical history. Atherosclerosis is the buildup of cholesterol and triglycerides in the arteries (plaque) and can occur even in small blood vessels throughout your body. You are probably most familiar with the blockage of a coronary artery resulting in a heart attack, but plaque can also cause blockages in your carotid artery or other arteries in your brain, potentially leading to a stroke if oxygen-rich blood can't get to a site because of the blockage. Or the lipids may narrow an artery or vein, making you more susceptible to a stroke from a blood clot. Cholesterol buildup can cause blockages in your femoral artery, which can trigger severe pain when you try to walk or even at rest. This type of blockage will interfere with the blood flow to your entire leg and can lead to infections, including gangrene.

Cholesterol is the main component in the plaque, and it is primarily oxidized LDL cholesterol that causes problems. Triglycerides and their metabolic by-products are also involved in this process. The proteins in HDL are packages that clean up cholesterol in your bloodstream and deliver it to the liver to be eliminated. Elevated triglycerides depress HDL levels, resulting in higher LDL-cholesterol and more plaque. Again, it's not just the large arteries that can get cholesterol deposits. Your eye doctor may be able to see cholesterol crystals in the back of your retina, which may be related to risk for age-related macular degeneration. Cholesterol can also block the small blood vessels in sex organs and lead to erectile dysfunction or to lower responsiveness.

Blood glucose is an important number to know for your heart, especially since elevated glucose can be an early warning sign of metabolic syndrome. If caught early, metabolic syndrome and higher blood sugar (elevated glucose) can often be managed by lifestyle changes in what you eat and your activity level. These lifestyle changes will have benefits for your health even beyond your heart. Your blood glucose level should be under 100 (5.6 mmol/L) to be considered healthy. (Being closer to 80 would be perfect.) If your glucose is between 100 and 125 (5.6 to 7.0 mmol/L), you are considered to have prediabetes, which is a component of metabolic syndrome.

Blood pressure indicates how your heart is functioning to move blood through your arteries and veins. Elevated blood pressure is an indicator that your heart is having to work harder than it should in order to move blood around your circulatory system. If your blood pressure is mildly elevated, you may be able to reverse it through changes to your diet (especially with the DASH diet) and adding regular activity that gets your heart beating a little faster, to improve your entire cardiovascular system.

High Blood Pressure

To better understand your blood pressure health at the start of this program, let's look in greater detail at what some of these conditions look like and how they are assessed. The 2017 blood pressure guidelines from the American Heart Association (AHA) and the American College of Cardiology, generated by the Joint National Committee on Prevention, Detection, Evaluation and Treatment of High Blood Pressure (JNC8), have the following blood pressure categories:

Classifications of Blood Pressure (United States)			
Blood Pressure Categories	Systolic Blood Pressure (Top Number) in mm Hg		Diastolic Blood Pressure (Bottom Number) in mm Hg
Normal (desirable)	Less than 120	and	Less than 80
Elevated	120–129	and	Less than 80
Stage 1 Hypertension	130–139	or	80–89
Stage 2 Hypertension	140 or higher	or	90 or higher

Table 2. *Classification of blood pressure AHA, ACC, JNC8, 2017*

Surprisingly, someone who has normal blood pressure at age fifty-five still has a 90 percent risk of developing hypertension at some point in their lifetime. However, while this is common, it is not a normal, healthy part of aging. There are populations in the world where blood pressure stays in the healthy range for their whole lives. And that is the goal here, too. We want to have all the blood pressure benefits of the DASH diet and all the heart-protective benefits of the Mediterranean diet. We want to stay healthy for our whole lives.

Stage 1 hypertension can be treated with lifestyle changes. Along with exercise, reaching and maintaining a healthy weight, the DASH diet and the Mediterranean diet are both recommended for optimal blood pressure. So, if these diets are so beneficial, why don't doctors recommend them more often? Unfortunately, many physicians think that taking a pill may be easier for their patients than changing their eating and exercise habits. We are going to change that perception.

Let food be thy medicine.—Hippocrates

Please *don't* think of food as medicine. Food is to be enjoyed. If a healthy diet feels like you are taking medicine, you are unlikely to enjoy it or want to keep following it. Enjoy the wonderful variety of food on the Med-DASH program, which may eliminate your need for medicine to control blood pressure.

Foods that are good sources of fiber, calcium, potassium, protein, and unsaturated fats are associated with improved blood pressure. Fortunately, the Med-DASH plan is rich in these key nutrients. By focusing on the important foods to include, you will easily be getting the right minerals, vitamins, antioxidants, and anti-inflammatory compounds to help you reach and maintain healthy blood pressure.

Atherosclerotic Heart Disease

Throughout your life, your initially clean arteries are gradually developing plaque that can eventually create a blockage in a vein or artery. As the result of autopsies done on service members during the Vietnam and Korean Wars, even young men of eighteen or nineteen were seen to have the beginnings of plaque buildup in their arteries. In servicemen killed in the Korean War, 77 percent had atherosclerosis (plaque), while 45 percent of Vietnam War casualties had plaque.

Today the medical profession is much more aggressive in monitoring and treating elevated cholesterol and other heart disease risk factors. Fewer people are smoking. Service members killed in combat today have much lower levels of plaque, with only 8.7% showing blockages.[4] Statins are standard therapy for elevated cholesterol for everyone. They substantially reduce LDL cholesterol but can also lower HDL cholesterol, the "good" cholesterol. It has been shown that statins reduce the risk of heart attack even more than just the reduction in LDL would suggest. Statins have a side benefit of lowering systemic inflammation, which provides additional benefits. And we can get many of these same benefits and more from diet and lifestyle changes. If we can't avoid the statins altogether, we can at least do everything we can with diet and activity to minimize the dosage we need to take.

If lowering cholesterol is as simple as taking a pill, isn't that enough? Actually, it would be even more beneficial to have your HDL cholesterol be high, at least over 60, while at the same time having your LDL cholesterol be as low as possible. Depending on your personal medical history, you should probably have an LDL level less than 100; if you have diabetes or have had a heart attack, your doctor will want you to be under 70. Although these guidelines are not as cut-and-dried as they used to be, they are most likely the standards that your doctor will use. And while statins lower cholesterol, they do nothing for triglycerides. Fortunately, the Med-DASH plan will cover all the bases, augmenting your medical treatment for elevated lipids (cholesterol and triglycerides) with a diet that also promotes heart health, including helping to lower bad cholesterol and triglycerides and increase good cholesterol.

The first step in developing plaque is a small buildup of fats (mostly LDL cholesterol) on the surface of artery walls.[5] This initial step can start to happen as early as childhood and adolescence. Factors that can speed this process include smoking, hypertension, diabetes, obesity, and genetics. The LDL can become oxidized and contribute to mild inflammation of the artery lining. Inflammation is a factor in making these deposits stickier, thus attracting more buildup. Later in the process, a thin fibrous layer will cover the plaques. These layers can rupture, exposing the fats and cholesterol, and potentially creating pieces that can plug an artery, known as thrombosis. In many cases, the rupture heals and becomes the base for a larger deposit of plaque. Sudden cardiac death can result when there have been multiple cycles of rupture and healing. Calcium is also a component in these plaques. New research is suggesting that calcium from supplements may be associated with increased risk for heart disease.[6] However, a diet that is rich in naturally occurring calcium, like the DASH diet, seems to be protective for heart disease as well as bone health.

When we measure the effectiveness of statins, we especially look at LDL. Cardiologists have found that the LDL reduction provides a window into evaluating the amount of plaque reduction. For example, if LDL is lowered from 160 to 100, that would reflect a significant reduction in plaque, therefore a big improvement in lowering cardiovascular disease (CVD) risk. Statins also seem to stabilize the remaining plaque and reduce the likelihood of rupture. In as little as four months, statins can reduce the risk of potentially life-altering consequences such as heart attacks, strokes, and TIAs (transient ischemic attacks, or mini strokes). This seems to result from a combination of lowering LDL and reducing inflammation.

The benefit of statins is persistent in reducing heart disease risks, even long after discontinuation of treatment (which I am not encouraging anyone to do). On the negative side, however, the use of statins is associated with increased risk for developing type 2 diabetes, particularly in women, the elderly, and people with a strong family history of diabetes.[7] It is to your benefit to make lifestyle changes to minimize the statin dosage you need.

Red Wine

Wine is typically consumed with meals in the Mediterranean area. The red wine in the Mediterranean diet appears to reduce the risk of plaque rupture, although just in the short term. It is rich in antioxidant and anti-inflammatory properties. You can get much of the same benefit with red grape juice.

HDL cholesterol can be thought of as a sponge that that helps to soak up cholesterol to help keep our arteries clean. If your HDL level is high, you have a good capacity for reducing LDL cholesterol, which, left untreated, can plug heart arteries. The whole-food, plant-focused Med-DASH plan helps you maintain an HDL level as high as possible. A diet high in refined carbs, sugar, and alcohol is more likely to produce higher levels of triglycerides. These fats are packaged in chylomicrons, which unfortunately have the

Controlling Triglycerides

- Avoid processed carbs and foods with added sugars, and limit juice.
- Drink alcohol only in moderation.
- Exercise to help your body process blood sugar better. Your muscles will respond better to your natural insulin and burn more glucose as fuel.

capability to soak up some of the cholesterol from HDL, shrinking them and lowering HDL, which is the opposite of what we want.

When your blood sugar is under control, you won't make extra triglycerides from excess glucose. Cardiovascular (aerobic) exercise helps with a whole host of interrelated problems, including excess belly fat, high blood pressure, prediabetes, and heart disease. In the next section, you will learn a lot more about this relationship.

Metabolic Syndrome: Prediabetes, Hypertension, and Heart Disease

We want to stay healthy for our whole lives. One of the most common and devastating conditions that can ruin our health is metabolic syndrome. This is a particular interest of mine, because on one side of my family, almost everyone has it, so I am also at high risk. It is a combination of at least three diseases: prediabetes or type 2 diabetes, high blood pressure, and undesirable levels of cholesterol and triglycerides, and excess weight around the waist. Fortunately, the Med-DASH plan addresses each of these problems.

It is possible to manage or even reverse metabolic syndrome. In order to understand how to do that, it is important to understand what metabolic syndrome actually is, and how it gets started. (A syndrome is a disease where you do not need to have each of the symptoms to be diagnosed.) At some point in our lives, we might become a little overweight. Perhaps we are not very physically active, and we might be eating too much processed food, especially starchy and added-sugar foods, and foods high in saturated fats. Initially, our body will make extra insulin to keep blood sugar under control. But at some point, our muscles become even less sensitive to insulin (this is called insulin resistance), and we start to wear out our ability to produce enough, leading to higher-than-normal blood sugar. The excess blood sugar causes you to gain extra weight around your waist, which further deteriorates blood sugar control. At this point, you could be diagnosed with prediabetes or diabetes. Our blood pressure gets higher than desirable. The high blood sugar causes triglycerides to increase, which lowers our HDL cholesterol. Each of these symptoms on its own is bad, but when they all happen at the same time, they can be especially problematic. And they can cause additional diseases such as kidney disease from high blood pressure or high blood sugar, fatty liver disease from excess triglyceride production, and nerve damage and pain from high blood glucose. Think of your diagnosis as your early warning, so that you can reverse it.

Metabolic Syndrome, Diagnostic Criteria

Symptoms (3 or more of the following)	American Heart Association/ American College of Cardiologists[8]	International Diabetes Federation[9]
Waist circumference	40 inches or more for men, 35 inches or more for women	Depends on ethnic criteria
Fasting blood glucose	100 mg/dL or greater, or receiving treatment for diabetes	5.6 mmol/L or greater, or being treated for diabetes
HDL (high-density lipoprotein) cholesterol	Less than 40 for men, less than 50 for women, or being treated for low HDL	Less than 1.03 mmol/L in men, less than 1.29 mmol/L in women or being treated for low HDL
Triglycerides	150 mg/dL or higher, or being treated for high triglycerides	1.7 mmol/L or higher, or being treated for high triglycerides
Blood pressure	Elevated blood pressure (greater than 130/85 mm Hg) or being treated for hypertension.	Systolic BP greater than 130 mm Hg and/or diastolic greater than 85 mm Hg, or being treated for elevated blood pressure

Table 3

Metabolic syndrome (and its related sister, polycystic ovary syndrome), unfortunately, is a widespread modern condition. The outward sign is an out-of-proportion waist size, often referred to as an "apple" body shape, or android obesity. The hidden signs are any of the following: elevated fasting blood sugar, elevated blood pressure, low HDL cholesterol, and high triglycerides. Almost one-third of adult Americans have diagnosed or undiagnosed metabolic syndrome. It is a warning sign that you are at elevated risk for heart attack, stroke, and type 2 diabetes. Fortunately, each of these conditions is improved with the Med-DASH program. Using the optional Med-DASH jump-start plan in this book (see page 109) will help you go a long way toward shrinking your waist size, an easy, visible way to evaluate whether you are taking the right steps to help control this condition.

PCOS

Polycystic ovary syndrome (PCOS) is very similar to metabolic syndrome in its presentation. However, it adds extra problems, such as difficulty conceiving and excess production of androgens. While it is a complex problem, the components related to metabolic syndrome (elevated glucose, excess abdominal fat, elevated triglycerides, low HDL, and elevated blood pressure) will respond to the Med-DASH plan to reduce or manage these symptoms.

Women and Heart Disease

While we tend to think of heart attacks as being primarily a concern for men, did you know that heart disease is the number one cause of death in women, too? Nearly one in three women will die of heart disease. That is more than those who die from all types of cancer combined.

Women's heart attack symptoms may be quite different from those of men. Chest pain or pressure are the most common symptoms for both men and women. However, women are more likely to experience shortness of breath, back or jaw pain, or nausea and vomiting as their primary symptoms, and may not recognize these as possible symptoms of a heart attack. Early treatment is critical to recovery. Even today, with all the education about heart health in women (such as the Go Red for Women campaign), women tend to get diagnosed later after the onset of symptoms. Fully two-thirds of women will never fully recover from a heart attack.[10]

How the Mediterranean and DASH Diets Help Keep You Healthy

One of the key ways the Med-DASH plan helps you lower your cholesterol is by reducing saturated fats. We can choose lean meats and poultry when we have animal proteins. (Beans are good protein sources and do not contain saturated fats. Additionally, their fiber helps to reduce absorption of cholesterol and fats during digestion.) Avoiding processed foods can limit exposure to trans fats and palm oil, which are very unhealthy for your heart. Both of these fats have been used to make processed foods, such as crackers and cookies, crispier. The primary fat in palm oil is palmitic acid, which is a saturated fat and readily used by the body to make cholesterol.

Reducing cholesterol that comes from food may be beneficial for treating heart disease, but it is not as important as reducing the amount of saturated and trans fats you consume. We normally consume over 100 times more of these fats than we do dietary cholesterol. Limiting saturated and trans fats has a huge payoff.

While many physicians still tell their patients to adopt a low-fat diet, reducing fat intake is actually counterproductive for heart disease and is no longer part of the lifestyle recommendations from

Sad, but True

Taking artificial trans fats out of foods has been a great idea—until the food industry found a way to replace one bad fat with another. The palm oil that has replaced trans fats in most processed foods is highly saturated and likely to cause higher blood cholesterol. Currently, the United States does not allow any artificial trans fats to be used in food products, but when it comes to harmful fats in processed foods, we aren't out of the woods yet.

the American College of Cardiology and the American Heart Association (AHA). You want to reduce harmful fats, not the beneficial ones. If you limit intake of all fat, it typically gets replaced by processed carbs, which can cause your body to make more cholesterol and more triglycerides. That is not heart healthy. From the AHA Presidential Advisory: "replacement of saturated fat with mostly refined carbohydrates and sugars is not associated with lower rates of CVD and did not reduce CVD in clinical trials."[11]

So how do you avoid refined carbohydrates, extra sugar, and harmful fats? Don't shy away from anything that has a higher fat content—just try to cut down on foods that contain palm oil or coconut oil. Healthy fats, such as those in avocados, nuts, and olive oil, should not be off-limits to you—and they aren't off-limits on the Med-DASH food plan. In addition to allowing you to enjoy foods that contain helpful fats, the Med-DASH plan has a built-in safety net to help your body process fats. It is super rich in plant foods that are high in fiber. Soluble (or viscous) fiber is great for trapping dietary cholesterol and fats during digestion, and not allowing them to be absorbed. Some of the best sources include beans, oats, barley, apples, pears, orange, berries, stone fruits (peaches, cherries, plums), and many vegetables.

The high levels of antioxidants found in plant-based foods are very beneficial for heart health because they reduce the body's ability to oxidize cholesterol. It is oxidized LDL cholesterol that is associated with creating plaque and potential blockages. Having a diet rich in antioxidants helps reduce this risk. Antioxidants also help reduce inflammation, which is an initiator for the components of metabolic syndrome. In addition to fruits and vegetables, onions, garlic, tea, and chocolate are also rich in antioxidants. High flavor and high health benefits!

The Mediterranean diet and the DASH diet have each been shown to be associated with lower risk for developing type 2 diabetes, which is a key component of metabolic syndrome.[12] Reducing processed foods enhances the risk reduction. Reaching and maintaining a healthy weight is also very beneficial for reducing risk of heart disease. Fortunately, the Med-DASH plan is very satisfying and filling, making it much easier to avoid overeating. Later, we will cover this in detail.

It's So Easy

You may have tried to eat healthfully before and either found it too difficult to sustain or never got the results you were expecting. It's time to expand the possibilities in your life. Have protein and fats to satisfy hunger more easily and longer, while also keeping blood sugar on a more even keel. This is the opposite of the old food guidelines, which had dieters eating foods stripped of precisely the nutrients that are filling and satisfying, making those foods less satisfying. This is what was wrong with the high-carb, low-fat/low-protein diet plans. Everyone became fatter precisely because these plans led to overeating. I am going to present a program that will improve your health and be easy to follow. You will love the food, and at the same time, it will help keep your hunger and cravings from overpowering your new eating plan.

The Med-DASH Plan to Curb Cravings and Keep You Satisfied

By choosing a diet without lots of processed carbs, you can avoid blood sugar rushes and subsequent crashes. The Med-DASH plan allows you to be satisfied without overeating. After so many years of following high-carb, low-protein/low-fat plans, you will find it much easier to achieve and maintain your desired weight.

- Sugar cravings are reduced when you can avoid the blood sugar roller coaster triggered by diets high in processed carbs. Foods high in processed carbs can cause a blood sugar rush followed by a crash, which then leads to more cravings.
- The plan encourages healthy protein-rich meals and snacks. Protein (either plant or animal protein) is digested more slowly than processed carbs and can get turned into glucose to keep blood sugar from dropping too low, thus providing energy when you have less sugar in your bloodstream (about an hour after eating). This satisfies hunger.
- Avoiding surges in blood sugar helps lower triglycerides.
- A fiber-rich diet helps slow digestion and the absorption of carbs, making it easier for your body to control blood sugar.
- Heart-healthy fats improve satiety at the end of a meal or snack, and keep you feeling full longer.

CHAPTER 3

The New Philosophy for Reaching and Maintaining a Healthy Weight for the Rest of Your Life!

This is new; this is real. Eat foods that fill you up. Eat foods that are satisfying. Everything follows from this.

Our goal is not weight loss. Our goals are losing excess body fat and maintaining muscle while eating in a way that makes us healthier.

The foundation of both the DASH diet and the Mediterranean diet is plant foods. Everywhere around the world where people lead healthy lives to an advanced old age, they consume mostly plant foods. Fruits and vegetables are full of water, so they are very bulky and filling, which has been associated with helping people moderate how much they eat without even trying. Add to that foods that are more likely to quench your hunger, and you'll naturally stop before overeating. The fact that these foods happen to be extremely rich in vitamins, minerals, and antioxidants is a huge part of how they keep you healthy. We don't count calories on this plan; we count food servings from the various food groups. You won't see a rigid prescription for calorie goals, and you won't see calories listed on our recipes or meal plans. Instead, you simply eat a variety of foods from the different food groups. Real foods. Eat to be satisfied and comfortably full. That is sustainable.

As a diet plan, the Med-DASH eating pattern is all about health. Weight loss is an important side benefit (if that is your goal). You will not feel like you are on a diet. This may be confusing, but it is so much more mentally healthy to not focus on your weight but on how the plan makes you feel. Are your clothes fitting looser? Do you feel more energetic? Have you been to the doctor and been told that your blood pressure is much better or your lipid levels are much improved?

Traditionally people have thought about diets as a way to lose weight. The Med-DASH plan is different. This is an eating pattern designed to be delicious and keep you healthier, and it can support weight loss, especially unhealthy abdominal fat. But how does this plan make us healthier? What have we been doing wrong that gave us these epidemics of obesity, cardiovascular disease (CVD), high blood pressure, and type 2 diabetes? Let's look at metabolic obesity, which may help us tie things together.

Metabolically Obese

Excess weight is a very important issue in most of the world. What do we mean when we talk about a healthy weight? It is a weight at which you don't have health problems associated with your weight. When the U.S. and World Health Organization (WHO) guidelines were developed about what it means to be overweight or obese, the standards were based on evidence that showed increasing health risks for higher body mass index (BMI). This doesn't mean everyone who is at a higher-than-desirable weight will have health problems. Many people are completely healthy at weight that would appear to be too high by BMI standards. But let's be clear. Being healthy *today* is one thing, but there is no guarantee about tomorrow. New research from studies following very large numbers of people for decades is casting doubts on the "obese but healthy" idea. People who are overweight are much more likely to develop CVD. Women who are obese but "healthy" are at a 40 percent higher risk of developing CVD and an 84 percent higher risk of developing a metabolic disease that corresponded to at least one of the conditions of the metabolic syndrome. This was reported from the Nurses' Health Study (NHS), which has been following over ninety thousand initially healthy women for forty-plus years.[1] In another study (which also included data from the NHS in the UK), obese men were 67 percent more likely to develop CVD and obese women were 85 percent more likely; both groups were more likely to develop it at a younger age than their counterparts with a lower BMI.[2]

BMI has its problems. It is based on a relationship between your weight and height. It is certainly possible for people to be very physically active and eat healthfully but still be classified as overweight or obese. Football players would be a perfect example. They might have a BMI that would put them in the obese category, but not be "overfat." And conversely, people can have a desirable BMI, but be totally inactive, eat lots of junk food, and be "metabolically obese." BMI is used by physicians in their evaluation of your health status because it is a very simple tool that gives a number for classification purposes. However, there are other ways to judge the impact of weight on health.

Evaluating whether someone is metabolically obese is much more complicated and can require lab tests and judgment on the part of the person's physician. Metabolic syndrome codifies metabolic obesity. One extremely easy measure that is used to evaluate metabolic syndrome is waist circumference. As we know, waist size is a marker that you are consuming (primarily) carbohydrates in excess of what your body can burn or store. Excess fat around the waist is associated with higher risk for high blood pressure, atherosclerosis, heart failure, fatty liver disease, type 2 diabetes, and some kinds of cancer, consequences that no one wants. All those outcomes are associated with metabolic disease.

Carrying extra weight around your waist is an indicator for when excess weight is associated with health risks and subclinical inflammation. BMI is not.[3]

Metabolic syndrome is the consequence of not changing lifestyle and eating habits when belly fat starts increasing. Your physician may notice that your labs and vitals show all or a few of these symptoms: high LDL cholesterol, high triglycerides, low HDL cholesterol, elevated blood pressure, and elevated blood glucose.

How Can This Be Avoided? What Can We Change?

Eating more plant foods is important. Avoiding empty carbs is an easy way to start reducing that excess abdominal fat. Instead, start making meals and snacks that are rich in fruits, vegetables, nuts and seeds, dairy, and additional protein-rich foods such as eggs, lean meat and poultry, seafood, and beans, along with heart-healthy fats. These foods will fill you up and keep you feeling satisfied longer.

A meal or snack high in starch and/or sugar will make you feel satisfied for a short time, but will tend to increase hunger later. These carbs can be quickly digested and absorbed by your body. These are called high glycemic index foods. You will get a sugar rush (since starch breaks down to 100 percent glucose,

Don't Lose Weight, Lose Fat!

If you are trying to lose weight, you only want to lose fat, not muscle. Losing muscle slows your metabolism. By choosing the right foods, you can maintain your muscle (or minimize muscle loss) and reduce fat in unwanted places, especially around your waist. Belly fat is unhealthy fat symptomatic of storing excess carbs in your abdomen, particularly if you are unable to process glucose as well as you should. The more fat you gain in your belly, the more likely you are to lose the ability to make enough insulin to clear glucose out of your blood quickly enough to avoid even more fat storage. And you could be on your way to type 2 diabetes. With the Med-DASH plan, you are going to learn how to reverse the fat storage machine of your abdomen and how to avoid losing the ability to produce sufficient insulin. In doing so, you will also lower your risk of heart disease, stroke, and some kinds of cancer. You will relearn how to eat. You will be more satisfied with each meal or snack, and cravings will become a thing of the past. Exercise (or movement, for a more positive image) will also be pleasurable; you won't be forced to join a boot camp or do three hundred crunches, lunges, or planks (unless of course that is something you really enjoy). You will choose healthy movement that is fun for you, activities that are pleasurable. Your heart will become stronger, your muscles and bones will become stronger, your everyday activities will become easier. You will utilize glucose during this activity, which will help avoid overtaxing your ability to produce insulin. That helps to ensure that you won't have excess glucose in your blood, ready to plump up your fat cells. Your exercise routine will work for you instead of against you. These are food and movement principles you can follow for a lifetime.

which is the blood sugar measured in people with diabetes). The sugar rush will trigger your body to produce insulin to control your blood sugar level. If your body is fit, you will respond well to the insulin and store the blood glucose in your muscles. If you don't respond well, your pancreas will pump out extra insulin, trying as hard as possible to bring the glucose under control. Unfortunately, your abdominal fat cells do respond well to insulin, so excess carbs can get stored there and get converted to fat. The liver will also try to store excess glucose, but after it reaches its capacity for storing glucose as glycogen, the liver will start turning glucose into fats. This leads to fat buildup in the liver and elevated triglycerides in your blood, both of which are unhealthy. It is very likely that the pancreas can overshoot its target while trying to keep glucose under control, and cause your blood sugar to get too low. The sugar rush and subsequent crash will lead to hunger and cravings for even more sugary or starchy foods.

If you eat a mixed meal, with high-fiber vegetables and/or fruit, protein-rich food, and some heart-healthy fats, you can avoid this sugar roller coaster. The high-fiber fruits and vegetables will digest slowly and release sugar into your bloodstream slowly. This won't overtax your ability to store glucose with just a moderate amount of insulin. The foods that provide fiber, protein, and fat will slow digestion, helping to keep you feeling full longer. The energy and glucose from these foods will be entering your bloodstream even slower than that from the fruits and veggies so you don't get that sugar crash. When we talk about the glycemic index of foods (the level that your blood glucose will spike to), we typically learn about individual foods. But nutrition scientists know that a mixed meal actually has a glycemic index based on the combination of foods and is much lower than for an individual high-carb food, based on the fiber, protein, and fat that slow digestion. No sugar crash, no excessive hunger, no cravings. You are full. An eating plan that gives your body what it needs so that you aren't at war with your appetite—what a concept![4] We aren't going to set rigid weight-loss goals or recommend a specific level of calories. You'll just eat a balanced, healthy diet.

Even more relevant than glycemic index is the glycemic load, the total amount of carbs that enter your bloodstream after a meal. You might have a food with a high glycemic index, but a small amount of sugar or starch. This would deliver a smaller glycemic load to your body. The glycemic load has been shown to support weight loss in people who were not in clinical trials, and free to choose their own foods and quantities.[5] The kinds of foods in the Med-DASH plan are consistent with having a total diet that is low in glycemic load. In the OMNICarb study, it was found that the DASH diet was effective regardless of the glycemic index of the individual foods.[6] Glycemic index in DASH did not affect markers of CVD risk or sensitivity to insulin, which would have indicated increased risk for type 2 diabetes. The high fiber in this plan, along with the balance of foods, shows that it is not necessary to evaluate either glycemic index or glycemic load with DASH, nor with Med-DASH.

Becoming more physically active is also a key component of the program. As you develop more muscle and become more aerobically fit, your body can burn more carbs, both when you are exercising and when you are at rest. After exercising you do need to replenish your energy level with a mixed meal or snack of high-fiber carbs, protein, and fat, just as we recommend throughout this book. Many people find that they eat more when they start a new exercise regimen. They think that because they are burning more energy, they can eat more. However, as we know, it is much easier to overshoot on calorie intake than it is to burn off the calories. You want to be more physically active in a way that you enjoy because it makes you feel great, not specifically as a way to burn off excess calories.

Med-DASH changes the focus from cutting calories and doing strenuous exercise to eating and moving joyfully. It is a plan you can sustain and embrace because it is satisfying on both counts.

CHAPTER 4

Surprising Benefits of the Med-DASH Plan

The Mediterranean and DASH diets have so many hidden benefits for the health of the whole body. These diets help reduce systemic inflammation, and risk of heart disease and stroke, type 2 diabetes, and certain types of cancer. They protect our bone health and kidneys, and may even be associated with a lower risk for depression.

Inflammation, Weight, and Chronic Disease

Subclinical inflammation is the beginning of many of our worst diseases, including heart disease, cancer, diabetes, and more. This inflammation is related to oxidative stress. Fruits and vegetables are the primary sources of antioxidants in our diets. Diets low in plant foods tend to be deficient in antioxidants, which can lead to oxidative stress. Many plant foods are rich in phytochemicals (plant chemicals), which help protect the plants themselves from diseases and can protect us as well. As you might guess, the Med-DASH

Phytochemicals

These are compounds made by plants that protect the plants from their environment. Most are not technically nutrients, but they do include powerful antioxidants, which can protect us as well. In the body, some of the carotenoids such as beta-carotene can be converted into vitamin A.

plan is super-rich in these plant compounds. It's so much nicer to eat some cherries or strawberries to reduce inflammation, as opposed to taking a pill.

Anyone who has rheumatoid arthritis (RA), which is also very sensitive to oxidants, can tell you about clinical inflammation. I have a neighbor with severe RA who wants desperately to avoid having to go on one of the biologic medicines, which can have severe side effects. She has discovered that a mostly plant-based diet, with fish, limited poultry, and almost no red meat, has done wonders for her inflammation. She does, however, get serious flare-ups if she has any meat. While she can draw an immediate connection between her diet and her symptoms, most of us cannot, and only find out about subclinical inflammation when we are diagnosed with a disease. Let's see if we can avoid that.

The Gut, Its Microbiota, and Inflammation

You're probably familiar with the phrase "Trust your gut": We are learning that there may be more truth to it than we thought. You've probably heard about serotonin, a feel-good neurochemical. It turns out that over 90 percent of your serotonin is produced in the intestinal tract, as opposed to in the brain (who knew?).[1] The bacteria in your gut is an important part of regulating how much serotonin is produced.

That collection of bacteria is called the gut microbiota, and discoveries about how it affects your health are coming in fast and furious. Some of the beneficial bacteria in your gut may produce fermentation products that help your body lose weight, whereas the unhelpful bacteria may produce end products that increase your likelihood of gaining weight. Some strains of good bacteria are linked to lower blood pressure, reduced inflammation, and lower risk for plaque buildup in your arteries. Many of these discoveries are still in the early stages, but they may help explain why food is more protective for health when consumed as a whole, rather than when the individual nutrients are consumed alone, such as with supplements. Fermentable fiber that supports beneficial bacteria may be a key part of the equation.

We've always known that fiber is good for your gut. Fiber is not digestible, but it can be fermented in the digestive tract, and that fermentation produces gases that actually nourish your intestinal cells. Some types of fiber, such as soluble fiber, nourish the good bacteria in your intestines, which have also been found to be important for maintaining health and a healthy weight. There is a (perhaps disgusting-sounding) procedure called a fecal transplant in which stool from a healthy person is transferred into an unhealthy person. Fecal transplants have also been used in obese patients, and studies have found that if the transplanted fecal matter comes from a vegetarian, it is more likely to result in weight loss in the person who receives it. Vegetarians have a beneficial mix of intestinal bacteria that may be the direct result of a diet particularly high in fiber.

Without fiber in the diet, the cells in your intestines may atrophy. The small intestine is where most of the nutrients from the foods you eat are absorbed by your body, and is actually much more powerful than you can imagine for nutritional health. The small intestine is quite lengthy, normally about 20 feet (6 meters) long, and has lots of folds to further increase its surface area. The villi, millions of small fingerlike projections lining the walls of the intestine, transport digested food (known as chyme) into your bloodstream. These villi have microvilli, which exponentially increase surface area for absorbing nutrients. Altogether the small intestines in a healthy gut have a surface area of nearly 200 square yards (about 200 square meters), allowing your body to efficiently absorb nutrients. This is a healthy gut. But without the right fiber, the villi can atrophy and become less able to transport nutrients into your bloodstream. Soluble fiber will ferment in the large intestines and produce gases, some of which are beneficial but some of which have no currently known benefits.

One of the most interesting new areas of exploration regarding inflammation and metabolic disease is of the bacterial population in the colon (large intestine). This microbiota is made up of ten times as many cells as we have in our whole body. These bacteria contain over three million genes, more than 150 times the number of genes we have in our whole bodies. Obviously, these bacteria must be very important for the proper functioning of the body's systems. As I mentioned earlier, transplanting fecal bacteria (my apologies for this image) from a vegetarian to an overweight person has been shown to induce weight loss. It is now believed that the beneficial bacteria in the transplanted stool are the result of having a plant-rich diet.

There is a direct relationship between the mix of bacteria in the gut and the amount of systemic inflammation in the body. Beneficial microbes can reduce inflammation, which is at the root of conditions that induce type 2 diabetes, high blood pressure, and atherosclerosis. The mix of bacteria will influence the production and absorption of harmful digestive by-products (such as lipopolysaccharides and peptidoglycans) that can increase your risk of developing type 2 diabetes. A beneficial mix of bacteria will produce more acetate, butyrate, and propionate, which are anti-inflammatory and maintain the health of the intestines by reducing permeability, thus protecting against harmful digestive by-products passing directly into the bloodstream. The relationship of a high-animal-fat diet and these diseases has been well-known for a long time, but the connection was not entirely obvious. Having a high-fiber diet leads to by-products of fermentation that are protective for the gut and the gut lining, and send beneficial anti-inflammatory agents into the bloodstream, by which they are carried directly to the liver. As a side benefit, some of these by-products, such as butyrate and propionate, may help with increasing satiety at the end of a meal.

The inflammation caused by an oversupply of bad bacteria leads to overproduction of certain immune cells, including mast cells, B-cells, macrophages, neutrophils, and T-cells, some of which can lead to the metabolic dysfunction that is associated with developing insulin resistance and to atherosclerosis.

Both prebiotic and probiotic solutions can promote better metabolic health by helping to reduce inflammatory digestive by-products. Diet also directly influences the mix of bacteria, and it can change quickly, in as little as five days. If you have seen the reports about how gastric bypass surgery results in a rapid reversal of negative metabolic processes, such as type 2 diabetes and blood pressure, the quick turnaround in health almost seems like a miracle. This is apparently associated with changes in the microbiome.[2] But without having to go through surgery, you can appreciate that this plant-focused diet change will be immensely beneficial for you as well. A diet rich in soluble fiber directly helps to reduce the metabolic inflammation associated with excess abdominal fat.

Another possible benefit of a healthy mix of bacteria in the digestive tract is that it can change the interaction of the neuro-transmitters produced in the gut and their communication with the brain. This appears to help reduce depression. It is well-known that metabolic dysfunction is associated with depression, but only recently was the link with the gut microbiome discovered.

Beneficial plant substances called polyphenols, in addition to being antioxidants, can also enrich the beneficial mix of the microbiota.[3]

Prebiotics and Probiotics

Prebiotics are substances that promote the growth of beneficial bacteria. They include fermentable fiber (most types of soluble fiber) and supplements such as fructooligosaccharides (FOS). A high-sugar or high-starch diet promotes the overgrowth of harmful bacteria. Prebiotics help support the development of a healthier mix of bacteria to reverse the problem.

Probiotics are beneficial organisms, such as the *Lactobacillus bulgaricus* and *Streptococcus thermophilus* microbes in yogurt and the *Lactobacillus acidophilus* and *Bifidobacterium bifidus* in acidophilus milk (milk fermented with these bacteria), each of which can help develop a healthy mix of intestinal bacteria. Beneficial bacteria can also be obtained through probiotic supplements.

Rich sources of polyphenols include fruits, vegetables, seeds, whole grains, and herbs, and beverages derived from plants, such as coffee, tea, cocoa, and wine (or grape juice for nondrinkers). You may have heard of flavonoids and non-flavonoids, including tannins, isoflavones (such as genistein from soy), flavonols (including quercetin), anthocyanins (which cause the purple-red color in many fruits and vegetables), lignans, and stilbenes (such as resveratrol from grapes). There is a mutually beneficial relationship between polyphenols and the gut microbiota. The bacteria help digest the polyphenols so that they can be absorbed, while the polyphenols help to support a health-promoting mix of bacteria. Some of the benefits that are attributed to polyphenols include helping to reduce the risk of cancer, heart disease, ulcers, and excessive tendency toward blood clotting, dilating blood vessels, modulating immune response, and pain reduction. Deriving these important benefits from polyphenols is dependent on having a healthy microbiota for their digestion and absorption.

Polyphenols	Examples	Good Food Sources
Flavenols	Quercetin	Onions, garlic, broccoli, tea, apples, wine
Flavenones and flavonones		Citrus fruits (oranges, grapefruits, lemons, etc.)
Flavones		Parsley, tea, chamomile, mints, citrus fruits, carrots, celery, olives, lettuce
Isoflavones	Genistein	Soy
Flavanols	Catechins	Fruits, tea, wine, chocolate
Anthocyanins		Blue-red fruits and vegetables, including blueberries, raspberries, strawberries, red cabbage, radishes
Phenolic acids		Whole grains, wine, berries
Stilbenes	Resveratrol	Red grapes, wine, strawberries, peanuts
Lignans		Fruits and vegetables, tea, coffee, whole grains, flax

Table 4

Inflammation and Heart Disease

Inflammation has been a hidden target for unifying many of our common problems. While it is not the be-all and end-all of health in and of itself, it is a contributor to poor health, which is easy to tackle with the Med-DASH plan. Delicious fresh fruits, including berries, plums, peaches, apples, and oranges, are rich in the anti-inflammatory plant chemicals. Colorful vegetables, including broccoli, red cabbage, tomatoes, bell peppers, and sweet potatoes, also are packed with these

Are Grapefruits Healthy?

People on certain medications are told to avoid grapefruit and grapefruit juice. Is this because grapefruits are unhealthy?
No. They are very healthy, like all citrus fruits. However, grapefruits contain a chemical that slows down the metabolism of certain medications, such as the statins used for lowering cholesterol. That means that the concentration of the medication will stay higher for longer than it should, which some people do not tolerate well. On the other hand, some medications need to be metabolized into an active form in the liver, and this slower conversion could prevent having sufficient drug activity as should be expected. If you aren't on one of these medications (your doctor, dietitian, or pharmacist should be able to tell you if you are), grapefruits are completely healthy for you.

protective compounds. Dark green leafy vegetables, spices, and herbs will also help reduce your risk for these diseases associated with inflammation.

People rarely hear about inflammation and heart disease from their physicians. A few years ago, everyone was checking C-reactive protein (CRP) levels along with cholesterol and triglycerides. However, insurance companies balked at another "unnecessary" test, and the practice mostly fell by the wayside. CRP is increased in inflammation, but it isn't specific for a particular disease. It could signal infection, cancer, heart disease, or several other issues.

But cardiologists know that inflammation is the beginning step in developing heart disease. And because overweight and obesity are at epidemic levels, weight is an important factor in increasing inflammation. In particular, excess abdominal fat is related to heart disease risk. We tend to think of an expanded waistline as particularly a male problem, and in fact researchers call it male pattern obesity. However, when women hit menopause and production of estrogen declines dramatically, they start storing fat around the waist and back. This corresponds with an increased risk for heart disease in women. Fat around the waist is metabolically active and leads to low-level inflammation throughout our body. The overproduction of immune cells outlined earlier in this chapter helps to promote the growth of cholesterol deposits in the heart arteries and, in fact, in blood vessels throughout our body.

We know from long-term studies that many of the key Med-DASH foods reduce the risk of heart disease. Previously we chalked all this up to lower cholesterol and blood pressure. But there is more to this story. Foods that are rich in antioxidants help protect your heart. It is oxidized LDL cholesterol that plugs up arteries. Antioxidants mostly come from plant foods that are rich in fiber to provide an extra boost to lower cholesterol.

A diet rich in fatty fish that are good sources of anti-inflammatory omega-3 oils is associated with a reduced risk of cardiovascular mortality. Recent studies of fish oil supplements have not shown the same advantages, although several older studies did show significant benefit. One of the largest was the GISSI-Prevenzione (Gruppo Italiano per lo Studio della Sopravvivenza nell'Infarto) trial, which showed a 40 percent reduction in cardiac sudden death and a 14 to 20 percent reduction in all causes of death by daily consumption of 1 gram of omega-3 fish oils per day for three and a half years. While we are now not so convinced about the supplements, fish as a whole food is beneficial for heart health. As in previously mentioned studies, most evaluations of supplements find that individual nutrients are not as beneficial as the whole foods from which they are derived. It is recommended that people have two or three servings (3 ounces or 90 grams cooked) of fatty fish per week (see Appendix D for good choices).

Oxidation and Disease Risk

Oxidation is a process of aging. It is the exact same process as when iron rusts. Oxidation makes our cholesterol stickier and more likely to cause buildups in our arteries. It can cause rancidity in fats in our body. It deteriorates the ends of our genes, called telomeres, which hastens the body's aging process and makes it more difficult to repair damaged cells. Oxidation of fats, primarily polyunsaturated fats, causes rancidity. In your body the oxidation occurs from free radicals, which are a reactive form of oxygen. And oxygen does react easily with nutrients in your body and can be an initiation step for some kinds of cancer. Oxidation also increases systemic inflammation in your body. (Systemic inflammation is usually low level but can initiate some processes that can lead to serious diseases.)

It's not just colorful foods that have antioxidant potential. For example, sulfur compounds that affect taste and scent in foods such as garlic, chives, and cabbage are very powerful antioxidants. Some chemicals in white foods, such as quercetin in potatoes, apples, and onions, have powerful antioxidant properties, and even may be related to slower aging.

Several vitamins and provitamins are powerful antioxidants. These include vitamin C, beta-carotene, vitamin E, and vitamin K. Vitamin C is found in most fruits and vegetables and of course, citrus fruits are especially good sources. Although it is water soluble, most other antioxidant vitamins are fat soluble, which means they are better absorbed when eaten with foods containing fats. Vitamin K is found in many leafy green vegetables and in vegetable oil; vitamin E is found in vegetable oils and in nuts and seeds; and beta-carotene is found in greens and orange-colored vegetables and fruits. The more of these compounds you consume from food sources, the better. And safer. With supplements you could consume excessive amounts, which can have the perverse property of actually promoting oxidation by transforming the antioxidant into an oxidant.[4] One of my professors was a lead researcher on a study that gave supplements of beta-carotene, vitamin E, and selenium (an antioxidant mineral) to Finnish men who were smokers, with the goal of reducing the risk of lung cancer. The study had to be stopped early because the researchers found more tumors instead of fewer. But it is very unlikely that you could consume excessive amounts of these compounds through eating real food as opposed to supplements.

Reducing the Risk for Cancer

Some types of cancer are based on genetic mutations, which may have occurred recently or many generations ago. But much cancer risk comes from lifestyle factors.

> ## Some Foods Rich in Antioxidants
>
> Apples, bananas, blueberries, broccoli, cauliflower, dark chocolate, garlic, grapefruit, kidney beans, lettuce, onions, oranges, peaches, peas, potatoes and sweet potatoes, raspberries, red and green cabbage, red grapes, red plums, red wine, spinach, strawberries, tomatoes

Smoking, eating a diet of junk food, excessive alcohol consumption, too much exposure to sunlight, and inactivity are all choices we make and can therefore change. Some people are very concerned about food additives and pesticides in their foods, but the type of foods being consumed is actually more of a problem than either additives or pesticides. A discussion of these issues is beyond the scope of this book. However, if you choose to avoid industrial pesticides, organic foods are readily available in most regions of the country. Even better is growing some of your fruits and vegetables at home, where you have control over how the food is produced. Many organic farmers' markets do a very good job of policing their food producers. Because the Med-DASH program is based on unprocessed or minimally processed foods, it is easy to avoid products with food additives.

Of course, a diet rich in fruits and vegetables is also rich in antioxidants. Reducing intake of omega-6 polyunsaturated fats, which are very susceptible to oxidation, is a great step and is encouraged in the Med-DASH plan. Although some wine can be part of the Med-DASH plan, overconsumption of alcohol is in no way part of this program.

Polyphenols from plant foods are capable of exerting antioxidant, anti-inflammatory, antiproliferative (halting the growth of cancer cells), and antiangiogenic (disrupting development of additional blood supply to cancer tumor cells) properties, all of which can have anti–cancer cell properties, or may help chemotherapeutic options become more effective. (Although it should be noted that oncology radiologists recommend against taking antioxidant supplements while patients are undergoing radiation therapy for cancer, because they will counteract treatment.)

Earlier in this chapter, we talked about how the Med-DASH plan helps to lower inflammation, which can help promote weight reduction, especially abdominal fat loss. This, in turn, reduces the risk of insulin resistance, elevated blood sugar, and type 2 diabetes. There are two ways that this reduces the risk for cancer. Higher-than-normal levels of insulin (a hallmark of insulin resistance) and excessive blood glucose both can feed the growth of cancer cells. And abdominal fat is capable of making estrogen, which can fuel the growth of some types of cancer, including the most common kind of breast cancer and some gynecological cancers. Some of the polyphenols listed earlier can act as naturally occurring selective estrogen receptor modulators (SERMs), which are used to reduce the likelihood of recurrence of breast cancers that are estrogen sensitive.[5] I also will note that the use of statins is associated with reduced likelihood of breast cancer recurrence, most likely via reduction of inflammation. However, statins are associated with increased risk for type 2 diabetes in postmenopausal women, with the risk increasing as the dose increases. Minimizing the medication dose you need via dietary changes is very helpful for avoiding potential negative consequences.

Keeping the Pancreas and Liver Healthy

The pancreas is the source of insulin, which helps regulate blood sugar. When you are young, your body responds easily to a high influx of sugar into the blood. The pancreas pumps out insulin, which helps to move glucose into your muscles to provide energy for activity. As you become older and if you also become more sedentary, your muscles stop responding as well to insulin.

Glucose is primarily stored in the muscles and secondarily in the liver, which is the primary reservoir for glucose that helps prevent blood sugar levels from dropping too low. Glucose is stored in the liver as glycogen, which is actually a human-produced form of starch. If your blood sugar drops too low, the hormone glucagon gets produced by the pancreas. It is used by the liver to break down glycogen into glucose, which the liver then pumps into the bloodstream to keep glucose from dropping dangerously low. Glucagon can also help initiate making glucose using amino acids (from protein), glycerol (from fats), and pyruvate and lactic acid (from glucose metabolism).

Many people develop insulin resistance (a component of metabolic syndrome) as they age. This is usually the result of a sedentary lifestyle, although there is also a genetic component to how likely you are to develop insulin resistance (IR). It is estimated that about one-third of adult Americans have IR, so it is quite common. With IR, the muscles stop responding as well to insulin. Your body pumps out extra insulin, trying to keep the glucose under control. However, fat cells, especially abdominal fat, still respond very well to insulin, which results in excess glucose getting stored in fat cells (primarily around your waist). This glucose can then be converted to more fat. As we gain more weight around our middle, the condition is amplified, making it worse and worse. And some of that excess glucose gets stored as fat in our liver. Too much of that results in what is known as nonalcoholic fatty liver disease (NAFLD), which is currently at an epidemic level in Americans.

The liver can also push some of this newly created fat into the bloodstream, which increases the level of triglycerides. High triglycerides can be an early warning sign of impending type 2 diabetes.

They raise LDL cholesterol levels and can lower HDL cholesterol. Consumption of fish rich in omega-3 fats can help keep triglycerides at healthier levels. Having only moderate intake of alcohol also helps avoid excess triglycerides and reduces the risk of fatty liver disease.

Eventually, your pancreas is unable to produce enough insulin to keep glucose under control. Then your blood glucose levels rise to above a healthy level and remain elevated, even after you've fasted for eight hours. These elevated levels can show up in blood tests, and based on those results, your physician may diagnose you with prediabetes. If your fasting glucose level is over 126, your doctor will probably do additional testing to confirm whether you have type 2 diabetes.

Fortunately, you can reverse this type of diabetes or prevent it from developing as was demonstrated in the Diabetes Prevention Program study, sponsored by the National Institutes of Health.[6] The key tools for accomplishing this are to become more active and to avoid eating lots of refined grains or sugar. On the positive side, you want to include more high-fiber vegetable foods. The foods with soluble fiber (or viscous fiber) are foods that slow down the digestion and absorption of sugar into your bloodstream, which makes it easier for your body to keep blood glucose under control with moderate insulin production.

You and your physician will be looking for lower fasting glucose levels and lower A1c (a measure indicating how well glucose has been controlled over the previous three months, also known as glycated hemoglobin). If you have type 1 or type 2 diabetes and are taking insulin, be sure to consult your physician and/or dietitian before starting any new eating plan. If you are on a sulfonylurea (such as glyburide), you may find that the lower carbohydrate nature of this program may cause you to become hypoglycemic. Metformin is less likely to cause hypoglycemia, but you should still discuss your diet and activity changes with your physician or diabetes educator.

Ask if you should (or can) discontinue these meds or reduce your dosage prior to starting the Med-DASH plan or according to your regular monitoring. In particular, if you choose to do the jump-start option, your need for insulin or glyburide may drop significantly. Reducing your need for insulin is a good thing in the long run, since it can slow or reverse diabetes progression. Most endocrinologists support a diet low in refined carbs and added sugars, especially if you are following a plan that you can really sustain.

Activity helps your body burn excess glucose for energy and can help resensitize your muscles to insulin. Even people with type 1 diabetes can develop insulin resistance, which causes you to need higher and higher doses of insulin. Three of the key benefits of the Med-DASH plan are that it avoids foods that will give you a sugar rush, it may help you reduce excess abdominal fat, and it encourages regular physical activity to burn glucose and help your muscles become more sensitive to insulin. Improved sensitivity means that your need for insulin decreases, and in the case of type 2 diabetes, it may help you avoid or delay wearing out your ability to produce enough insulin.

A Young, Healthy Brain

A very exciting development in research on the Med-DASH plan showed that people who followed this eating pattern were less likely to develop Alzheimer's disease. The lessons learned from this study, entitled the MIND diet,[7] provide real promise for avoiding this dreaded disease. Separately, each diet has shown encouraging results for reducing the risk of dementia. Some of the key reasons may include improved blood pressure, less atherosclerosis, and less inflammation. The high level of antioxidants may also be very beneficial for brain health. The omega-3 fats in fish are beneficial for brain health in several ways, including cognition, brain development, and perhaps controlling depression, and the Med-DASH plan encourages two to three servings each week. Fish has been long known as "brain food," and now we know a little more about why that may be.

Muscle Power

Your body is as old as your muscles. Most people lose muscle as they age. The less muscle mass you have, the older your body is. The more you can preserve or increase muscle mass, the younger you will feel. Everything you do in your daily routine becomes much easier. Strength training is one of the most valuable and one of the most overlooked types of activity for maintaining your physical well-being. Another key element in maintaining muscle tissue is getting sufficient protein in your diet. As we get older, many of us do not consume as much protein as we need. As a percentage of total calories, we need proportionately more protein as we age (or as our body "doesn't age"). The Med-DASH plan will provide sufficient protein to help keep your muscles strong, assuming that you do your part and stay physically active.

The Framework: Your Bones

The DASH diet and the Mediterranean diet have both been shown to be protective for bone health. Surprisingly, it's not just the calcium these diets contain, although DASH includes many foods rich in calcium. Let's learn how this works.

You may have been told by your physician that you have osteopenia (lower than desirable bone density) or osteoporosis (low bone density that can increase your risk of a fracture from a simple fall). It is generally diagnosed by a DEXA scan, which shows how your spine and the top of your femur (the ball that goes into the socket of your hip joint) compare in mineral content in relation to those of healthy young people. It might seem like a hip fracture isn't that big of a deal, especially with the advent of hip replacements, but in fact for almost 30 percent of people, it leads to death within one year, as limited mobility can lead to quick deterioration of overall health. Osteoporosis can also lead to spinal compression fractures, which can be very debilitating and painful.

The traditional advice for people with osteopenia and osteoporosis has been to take calcium supplements. However, it has recently been found that these supplements do little for bone health without adequate vitamins D and K and may contribute to worsening the buildup of artery-blocking plaque. On the other hand, people who have diets rich in calcium are less likely to have heart disease.

This is another example of how supplements with isolated nutrients are less beneficial than consuming the whole foods rich in those nutrients. Having said that, many people do need vitamin D supplements. In the northern hemisphere, people living in areas north of Indianapolis, Philadelphia, and San Francisco cannot make enough vitamin D between September 21 and March 21, when the sun's rays are more indirect, even if they are in the sun frequently. Even during the times of the year when the sun is more direct, many people do not make sufficient vitamin D because they wear sunscreen to protect their skin. Drinking milk and eating yogurt fortified with vitamin D are very beneficial; these foods are a key part of the Med-DASH plan for controlling blood pressure and provide minerals that support bone health. The same fish that are rich in omega-3 fats are very good sources of naturally occurring vitamin D.

The newest studies on osteoporosis are looking at long-term consequences of eating patterns rather than on short-term calcium metabolism. Calcium supplements, even with vitamin D, do not appear to reduce the likelihood of hip fractures. Vitamin K may be protective, as research has shown that women who consume at least one daily serving of green leafy vegetables (a good source of vitamin K) are 50 percent less likely to have hip fractures than women who only consume one serving per week. Having sufficient but not excessive protein in your diet is also important for bone health.

You probably could guess that the DASH diet would be very good for bone health, since dairy plays such an important role in blood pressure benefits, but who would have expected the same from the Mediterranean diet? But that is exactly what has been found. Specifically, spinal bone density was stronger in women following a Mediterranean diet than in those consuming a more typical Western diet.[8]

One of the reasons that this benefit may occur is that plant-based diets seem to be very helpful for absorbing more of the calcium in our diet. Paradoxically, it seems that the lower your calcium intake, the better your body becomes at absorbing dietary calcium. Increased physical activity that is typical in Mediterranean countries is also beneficial for bone health. It is very common for people in the region to take an early evening stroll for an hour or two every day. And walking is known to help maintain bone mineral density.

The activity level recommended with the Med-DASH program helps to maintain bone health. The best exercise for bone health is any that involves putting some stress on your bones, such as running or walking, jumping rope, strength training, and even yoga, each of which can help preserve or even increase bone density. Although putting stress on your bones may seem like the wrong thing, it actually encourages your bones to become stronger, similarly to how training with weights strengthen your muscles.

CHAPTER 5

Want Different Results?
Do Things Differently!

You may have some stubborn habits that are hard to give up. First, we are going to crush several dieting myths and break old bad habits. You will change how you eat. As hard as it may seem to give up treasured ideas and routines, you do want different results, so you will need to do things differently. You want to sweep out the concepts that can hold you back. All of us have been struggling with misinformation for so long that we hardly know what to eat. And perversely, it is precisely the people who have been trying to eat healthfully who are often the most confused about what to eat. We have all felt like we have been slung from one direction to another when it comes to nutrition advice. But fear not. We will enthusiastically embrace the true and enduring path to better health and well-being. And the good news is that a lot of delicious, decadent foods will actually be going back onto your "To Eat" list.

We are not going to focus on weight loss per se. Instead, we will emphasize relearning how to eat. You will eat for pleasure. Instead of limiting what you eat, you will make positive choices about what to include. Deprivation just leads to cravings and causes you to feel bad about how you are eating and the choices you make. Instead, we will focus on what to embrace, not what to exclude. So much more positive. You will choose foods that make you feel good, foods you can enjoy. A plan flexible enough to have room for your favorites, without making you feel like you are "cheating." That is gone! Banish the very idea of "cheats." That is not part of any emotionally healthy plan. And your emotions are just as important as physical health in this plan.

Health Myths, Busted!

There are health and nutrition myths that get you off track and prevent you from actually becoming healthier. Many of them even have been and continue to be promoted by health professionals and mainstream media. Some come by word of mouth. But clearly, if we want different results, we need to reexamine our underlying beliefs about the things that will make us healthier, including how we eat. Let's dispose of the myths.

"I know my body, I know what I need." (Or "I know my body, and I'll know if I have to go to the doctor.") Really? You can't sense if you have high cholesterol, high blood sugar, or high blood pressure. These are mostly silent diseases, and potentially silent killers. You can't sense if your bones are strong enough. This is another silent killer, since the immobility from hip fractures can lead to death within one year for about 30 percent of people. There are more. I had a very dear friend who put off dealing with symptoms for a year, even though her friends strongly urged her to see her doctor. Unfortunately, by the time she saw a doctor, they found stage IV cancer. Don't get fooled into thinking that you know your body and that everything is okay. While the

Med-DASH program is super health-promoting, it's not enough on its own to ensure good health. You are going to find key tips for optimal health here, but you still need to get regular checkups, because you can't know which silent killers are trying to destroy your health and your quality of life.

"I know what I have to eat, I just choose not to do it." If your eating plan or diet is too hard to follow or doesn't fit into your lifestyle, perhaps it is off track. And if it doesn't include the foods you really love, how can you stay with it? Perhaps you don't know as much as you think about what to eat, and have thought that you have to be very restrictive. If you are looking to improve on what you are doing to get better results, you really need to be open to change and new ideas on diet.

"I watch my calories, but I'm not able to lose weight." When you follow the guidelines for the Med-DASH program, you don't need to watch calories. You will be pleasantly satisfied without overdoing calories.

"I do boot camp [or run 5 miles, do 200 crunches, etc.] every day, but I can't lose weight." Sometimes, when people start exercising heavily, they either increase their eating or are so fatigued after exercising that they become less active later in the day. In fact, I have seen this when counseling Olympic-caliber figure skaters. After hours of practice, some adopted slug behavior and then found weight creeping on, even while they restricted what they ate. And not all exercise will give you the results you are seeking. Doing 200 crunches or lunges will not provide much benefit for the amount of tedious effort you're expending, and can make you hate to exercise rather than promoting a healthy, active lifestyle.

"My friend ran marathons but had a fatal heart attack at fifty. So why bother?" You may know someone who has taken perfect care of himself, but ended up having a heart attack much too young. Conversely, some people take poor care of themselves and live long, healthy lives. But we don't know which category we fall in, until it's too late. Most of us will get a huge benefit from having healthier habits. Our goal is to be as healthy as possible, for as long as we live.

Dangerous Nutrition Myths

We don't just have misconceptions about how to be healthy, but also about what to eat. So let's throw out what we don't need from the counterproductive nutrition advice of the past. We will rid ourselves of the dangerous nutrition myths of the last twenty-five years!

Eat 11 or 12 servings of grains each day.

It's hard to imagine food guidelines recommending that someone should eat eleven or twelve slices of bread every day. But that's exactly what we got with the Food Guide Pyramid from 1992. People joyfully piled on the carbs. Not beneficial whole grains, but plates heaping with pasta, endless bread baskets, and boxes of fat-free cookies. While Americans became more obese. Research has shown that foods that contain more moisture are more satisfying and filling. Bread? Very dry. Dense with calories. It's so easy to finish each refill of that endless bread basket, because we don't get full. Do you remember people eating whole boxes of cookies because they were fat-free? And yet they had the same amount of calories as the regular cookies and were higher in junk carbs.

Whole grains can be a very healthy part of the diet. But refined grains, without the fiber and stripped of most of the minerals, can become a problem, and are mostly empty calories. Your body quickly breaks down the fiber-less starch into glucose (which is our blood sugar), which then surges into your bloodstream. This may temporarily satisfy your hunger, but you will probably be hungry again in 45 to 60 minutes, when you get a sugar crash. Choosing mostly whole-grain foods instead of refined grains is more satisfying.

Juicing and smoothies are a great way to get fruits and veggies into your diet.

The proponents of juicing will tell you that your blender is a great way to help you incorporate lots of fruits and veggies, far more than you could normally eat, into your diet. Sounds great, but it doesn't work out so well for health, and it also misses the point: Whole fruits and veggies are beneficial precisely because they are filling. They naturally help you avoid overeating. That is a good thing. (More on this topic in chapter 6.) Fruits and veggies are a great source of antioxidants. Whipping air into them, unfortunately, neutralizes much of their antioxidant potential, wiping out the benefit. Fiber also takes a hit. Those whirring blades pulverize the fiber, making it virtually useless and thus crushing one of the key nutritional benefits of plant foods. In addition, if you have fruit in your smoothie, pulverizing it breaks down the cell walls along with the fiber, which will lead to a sugar rush, followed by a crash. Intact, whole fruit gets digested and absorbed more slowly, without triggering the sugar roller coaster.

Protein bars are great meal or snack replacements.

Protein or energy bars are great for athletes who need a concentrated, portable form of energy. If that's not you, eating protein bars can be counterproductive. They **are** a concentrated form of energy, and energy means calories. Sugar is the glue that holds most of them together. You will find that a Snickers bar has about the same nutrient composition as most energy bars. I personally would rather have the Snickers, and I wouldn't be fooling myself about its nutritional benefit. While protein is great to help satisfy hunger, you also want foods that contain lots of moisture to help quench hunger better and longer. Having a glass of milk with some berries or a peanut butter and jelly sandwich are both great, nutritionally balanced ways to replenish after exercise, or as an in-between-meal snack.

Small changes are best.

We've all heard that making small changes is a great way to develop new habits. However, if it takes a long time for you to see results, you may lose your motivation and move on without reaching any of your goals. For most of us, big changes that produce big results are powerful motivators. You just need to make sure that the changes are practical and fit into your real life. The jump-start plan in this book (see page 109) will give you big results through big changes and sets the stage for long-term success. Hundreds of thousands of people have adopted this strategy and love how they have been able to change their lives.

Americans eat too much protein.

The protein guidelines from the DRIs (Dietary Reference Intakes) are based on evidence for preventing starvation. However, for optimal health and maintaining or increasing muscle mass (which is related to your quality of life and metabolic rate), protein intake should be much higher. As a dietitian, early in my career, I was trained to calculate nutrient goals for weight loss by cutting all sources of calories proportionately. It turns out that this is a very bad idea. One of the keys to sustainable weight loss is to maintain protein intake at a level that minimizes muscle loss during weight loss. You know how everyone says it is so hard to maintain weight loss? With inadequate protein, a weight-loss plan will cause you to lose muscle mass, which slows your metabolism, and makes it very hard to keep the weight off. Is that your goal? Losing weight can be hard enough without self-defeating your progress by losing muscle and slowing your metabolism.

Weight loss is the goal of your diet.

Weight loss is *not* your goal. Sustainable weight loss is your goal (that is, if you need to lose weight). You only want to lose fat, not muscle. In the paragraph above, you learned about maintaining metabolic rate by maintaining muscle. You need to eat enough protein. To lose fat, we don't want to excessively restrict fat, however, because fats are critical for satisfying hunger. It's the empty carbs, the ones with no fiber and not much in the way of vitamins or minerals, that are the problem. Empty carbs aren't just sugar, but also include refined grain products, which are mostly starch. Occasionally they may still be referred to as complex carbohydrates (another holdover from the '90s). However, they aren't that complex for the body to break down. And they get broken down into 100 percent glucose. Gram for gram, starch produces more glucose than table sugar (sucrose). Sucrose only breaks down to 50 percent glucose (with the rest being fructose). Over time, excessive intake of starches can wear out your body's ability to produce sufficient insulin, which can lead to type 2 diabetes. Furthermore, any excess glucose your body doesn't need for quick energy gets stored in your fat cells, primarily in your belly fat. Excess weight around your middle isn't just a problem for how your clothes fit—it is associated with increased risk for heart disease, diabetes, high blood pressure, and some types of cancer.

It's in my genes to be heavy [or to have heart disease, or diabetes, etc.].

While family history of heart disease is a risk factor for your own personal heart health, there are things you can do to reduce your risk. Both the Mediterranean and DASH diets are proven to reduce your chances of developing heart disease. The same goes for genetic risks for type 2 diabetes and for being overweight. While your genetic code might place you at increased odds of struggling with these issues, we are going to minimize your risk. The healthy eating patterns of the Med-DASH plan will help you seize control of your future and not be destined to relive your family history.

Nobody needs to lose weight.

Who would have expected that weight loss would fall victim to political correctness and the "health at any size" movement? Certainly we do not want to promote fad diets that make us less physically healthy and the fat shaming that makes us less psychologically healthy. Yes, it is possible for people to be healthy and overweight. However, some things are not possible to wish away just to be "politically correct" about weight. Excess weight is associated with joint problems (osteoarthritis), sleep apnea, many types of cancer, gallbladder problems, decreased mobility, and fatty liver disease. And as you now know, excess fat around the middle (which can develop in people who are at a desirable BMI as well as those who are classified as overweight or obese) is associated with cardiovascular disease, type 2 diabetes, cancer, and more.[1]

The weight loss associated with the Med-DASH plan attacks the inflammation that accompanies excess mid-body fat. Empty carbs, such as those from foods high in added sugars and refined grains, feed the bad bacteria that can make your weight and health problems even worse, leaving you caught in an endless escalation of health problems and increasing weight. Having a diet that is packed with nutrient-rich plant foods, has sufficient protein, and is low in saturated and trans fats, while including heart-healthy fats to help make your meals satisfying, will make it easier to lose weight, thereby lowering inflammation and health risks.

You need to count calories to stay on track.

While research has shown that people who journal what they eat are more successful at reaching their health and weight goals, with this program, you do not need to track calories. Rather, you will track how many servings you eat from different food groups. Eating enough fruits, veggies, protein, dairy, etc., is key to getting all the benefits of the Med-DASH eating plan, especially since DASH is based on specific ranges of servings from the various food groups. The hidden benefit of this plan is that you will feel more satisfied with your meals and snacks, without fearing that you are going to overeat. You will develop habits that will take over and make it easy to follow the Med-DASH plan without thinking too much about it. So relax and enjoy the fabulous foods!

To lose weight, just reduce your calorie intake and exercise more to give a 500-calorie-per-day deficit.

Unfortunately, life isn't fair. It takes so little time to consume lots of calories and so much longer to burn those calories off. For example, a typical Thanksgiving dinner of 5,000 calories is easy to consume, but would take forever to burn off. For someone weighing 154 pounds (70 kg), walking 4 miles per hour for 2½ hours would only burn 900 calories, even though you have walked 10 miles. You can see that this is completely unfair and unbalanced. It's so easy to overdo calories, while it takes so long to burn them off. Furthermore, some people work out so strenuously that they become really fatigued and are more inactive later in the day. They go home or to the office after exercising and just sit. They may actually end up burning fewer calories during the day than before they started exercising. Or their appetite may increase, especially if they don't eat the right post-exercise foods to satisfy their hunger and replenish their nutritional needs. This is another example of life's unfair determination to make it hard to reach

The Countdown on Calories

Is a calorie a calorie? Almost all diet doctors will tell you that your weight is based on "calories in and calories out." They will tell you that the first law of thermodynamics states that, in a closed system, you can't make or destroy energy. (We measure energy by calories.) However, it has been misinterpreted to mean that the only key issues for weight loss are calorie intake versus calorie burning. But it is not that simple. First, the human body is not a closed system. Our metabolism is very complicated. Even our gut microbiome can influence how much of our food is digested and absorbed, and therefore how much energy we derive from it. Not all sources of calories are equal. Protein consumes more energy when it is metabolized than do carbs.[2] Furthermore, the old philosophy ignores that free-living people (i.e., those not cooped up in a metabolic lab) eat according to their own wishes. A large part of that has to do with how satisfying the food is, and how long it keeps you feeling satisfied.

your goals for health and weight, but it is one that can be overcome by the Med-DASH program.

Losing weight is just based on calories in, calories out.

It's not just "calories in, calories out." Yes, that's what we've been told. Even by prominent diet doctors and researchers. But it is not true. There is so much more to the story. It's the way food is digested, the way it is absorbed in the intestines, the metabolic consequences of your genetics and body type, the microbiota in your gut, and your muscle mass. It is a factor of the metabolic process of storing and burning fuel in your body. Perhaps you've always blamed yourself for not being able to reach a comfortable weight. It's time to stop. A fresh viewpoint will help you understand how to end your war with weight and make peace with your body.

All foods can fit.

This is my favorite one. It was so popular in the '90s. My own dietetic association adopted this as their slogan. And it is still bouncing around. The catch is that we all became fatter trying to fit it all in. How does this provide any direction for how we should eat? I love Snickers and chips. Should I make them the basis of my eating plan? Probably not. Instead of focusing on why we don't need to exclude certain food groups, perhaps the advice would have been more helpful if it had focused on what we should include or emphasize—so much more of an enlightening and positive message.

But it's healthy!

Lots of people think that if a food is healthy, they can eat as much as they want. For example, my husband will find a pint of blueberries in the refrigerator and finish it in one sitting. Or some people have several bowls of a whole-grain cereal because it's healthy. Yes, of course these foods are healthy, but you really want to have a *mix* of healthy foods. What could you include with the berries to avoid overdoing? Something with some protein, like yogurt. What would help you avoid bingeing on cereal? Perhaps topping it with some of those blueberries or some other favorite fruit. Fill the bowl with lots of milk, which is protein rich. The meal or snack will be more satisfying (and healthy) if it contains a variety of types of foods.

Eat Less, Move More (ELMM).

Just more of the same useless advice. Eat less of what? Everything? Vegetables? Fruits? Dairy? Nope. You want more of these bulky, filling, health-promoting foods. You want enough protein, you want satisfying heart-healthy fats, and you want less of the empty carbs. It's more important to know what to choose and what will satisfy hunger. As for exercise, there is almost no way to move enough to burn off excess calories. Yes, in general, we all do need to move more. However, certain kinds of exercise are more fun and more beneficial than others, so why not focus on the types with more of a payoff for boosting metabolism (which would not be crunches), making you stronger (which also would not be crunches), and making your life more active in general? Go dancing, walk in the park, go for a swim. But don't exercise to lose weight—exercise because it makes you feel better and more energetic, and actually makes your body younger.

The Time Is Now. Let's Start the Rest of Your Life!

Since we are so used to having short, pithy, albeit useless nutrition sayings, perhaps we can work with some that are actually true and helpful. Ones that can help you learn how to eat in a positive way for the rest of your life. Let's adopt some new nutrition slogans—helpful ones.

If you want different results, you need to do things differently.

Oops! This one is really hard for many people. It can be very difficult to give up all these myths that you were told would make you healthier. For some people, it's the smoothies or the protein bars that will be difficult to change. For others, it's adding foods with heart-healthy fats instead of always choosing fat-free foods. They may believe it will be impossible to survive without their old ideas, which have become the bedrock foundation of how they eat. If you are here to get different results and adopt a new way of eating, let's give it a try and move forward.

Eat to satisfy hunger and stay full longer.

We are going to learn about a new way of eating that will make it so easy to stay on track. You will love this new style of eating and will be amazed at how far off track all your old ideas were. I love it when readers complain that they have trouble eating all the foods included in a typical day on the Med-DASH plan. That happens when you have lots of veggies and fruits, eat enough protein, and avoid reduced-fat foods. People get full. When was the last time you heard this about a diet plan? Never?

Focus on what to include, not what to limit.

Traditionally, diet books have focused on what to avoid. Bad foods. Excess calories. Scrap that! How much more fun will it be to focus on what you want to include, not what you want to limit? What could be better than fresh foods? Delicious, beautiful food, with a Mediterranean overlay. Italy, Greece, Spain, southern France, Morocco, and the coastal regions of the eastern Mediterranean Sea. This is where the Slow Food movement isn't just a trend but a way of life. How fabulous to be able to enjoy the flavors of fresh foods and the region's herbs and spices! All your favorites. This is living!

Follow a lifelong eating pattern.

It is great to find a healthy eating plan. But what good does that do you if you can't sustain it for the long run, if you are hungry a half hour after you've eaten, if you or your family don't really like the foods on the plan, or if it doesn't fit into your lifestyle? The Med-DASH plan is going to change all that, right here, right now! Great-tasting, beautiful food. Satisfying meal plans.

Focus on Your Motivation

Taking care of your health can seem quite a challenge in a busy life. And it might seem like it would be okay to wait a few years until you really get concerned about it.

You might be thinking about this because your doctor issued a warning about what would happen if you didn't change your lifestyle. Or perhaps one of your relatives had an "event" such as a heart attack or stroke. You might see older people in your family who are physically incapacitated at too young of an age. You might just want to stay healthy for your kids and get them off on the right start with great habits. You might just want to feel great and be healthy for as long as you can.

There are all kinds of motivations for getting started on a new plan. But first, you need to think about what you are willing to do. If you set your expectations super high, you may disappoint yourself if you can't be perfect, quickly. If your goal is to add more cardiovascular (aerobic) activity to your day, you don't start by trying to run a marathon. Obviously, this would set you up for failure. But can you walk for 10 minutes? Or maybe a half hour? That would be a great start.

You want to set realistic expectations, which are achievable. Focus on your actions rather than the outcomes you are expecting. Can you add more vegetables to your diet? Sure! Can you have some yogurt as a snack? Sure! Can you spend 10 minutes walking today? Sure! Can you go to the grocery store and buy more fresh and frozen vegetables and fruits? Of course! These are practical steps you can take as you get started on this plan. By focusing more on the actions that you will take, you will find that this plan becomes much easier and less stressful than if you focus solely on your desired outcome.

In this book, you will learn strategies to make the Med-DASH plan work for your whole family. This plan will set the stage for your success. You will have meal plans that you can follow precisely or use as templates for your own food preferences. Whether you are a part-time or full-time vegetarian or a dedicated carnivore, you will find support for how you like to eat. You will learn what to keep on hand to make it easy to follow the Med-DASH program—how to stock up, how to do some prep work to make your week easier—and find recipes that are delicious as well as easy to make. Like to eat out frequently? Fear not. You will be able to maintain your lifestyle with our tips.

You are on to a new adventure. Fabulous food, good health, and desirable weight. All in one plan. Your Med-DASH program.

CHAPTER 6

The Big Three

Fats, proteins, and carbs are known as macronutrients, and they are the nutrients that provide calories. Each of them has been maligned at different times, but all three are essential, and we consume them in large amounts. But we need to clear up some misconceptions, and even ditch some bad ideas that have been part of the dietary guidelines, so we can choose wisely. Each of these nutrients has an important place in the Med-DASH plan, and we are going to find the balance among them that allows us to be healthy and keep a young body. Since we are focusing on whole foods instead of individual components, we are also going to learn a little about some of the non-caloric, non-macronutrient components that accompany these healthy foods.

The key DASH and Mediterranean diet foods are rich in nutrients and other components that help to make us healthy. We all know that vitamins and minerals are important for good nutrition. But you may not know as much about the other food components, such as fiber, phytochemicals and antioxidants, fats, and protein, that are equally important to our good health. Read on to learn more.

Fat Chance

After U.S. dietary guidelines were changed in the mid-1980s, people were encouraged to dramatically cut down on fats. We had fat-free dressings, fat-free cheese, fat-free cookies. All of it designed to reduce calories. Since fat is calorie-dense (containing 9 calories per gram instead of 4 calories like starch, sugar, and protein), it logically seems that this would help lower calories and make it easy to lose weight. Is that how it turned out? No. Since those guidelines appeared, the United States went from having 15 percent of adults being obese to 38 percent.

How could this happen? One of the benefits of fats is that they help you to feel full after a meal or snack; we call this satiety. And it is a very important concept in feeling satisfied with moderate amounts of food. This might seem like a no-brainer, when you consider how we react to food. And yet fat reduction was pushed as a way to avoid excessive intake of calories.

Another benefit of fats is that they help with the absorption of certain key vitamins, the fat-soluble ones, like vitamin A, vitamin D, vitamin E, and vitamin K. The very important antioxidants, carotenoids, are also fat soluble. They include beta-carotene (the orange in carrots and the provitamin converted to vitamin A in the body), lutein (a pale yellow in sweet corn, and found in especially high levels in spinach), lycopene (the red color from tomatoes), and zeathanthin (a red-orange compound found in high amounts in leafy green vegetables, among others). While the names of these phytochemicals are not important to remember, fruits and vegetables are rich in them, and they can have a significant impact on your overall health and well-being. You have long heard about the health benefits of antioxidant-rich foods, and now you know a little more about how they perform their magic. How sad that the old dietary guidelines emphasized low-fat eating, which reduces the absorbability of these key nutrients during digestion.

There are three main categories of fats, monounsaturated (MUFA), polyunsaturated (PUFA), and saturated fatty acids (SFA). (We will use the terms "fats" and "fatty acids" interchangeably, without making you take a chemistry lesson to fully explain it.) Saturated fats can be used by the body to make cholesterol, and are recommended to be consumed in small amounts. On the other hand, they are quite stable to oxidation, which means that they are unlikely to become rancid. Polyunsaturated fats include the heart-healthy omega-3 fats such as those in cold-water fatty fish, and omega-6 fats such as those in soybean or corn oil. The omega-6 fats are quite susceptible to rancidity, both in your kitchen during storage and in your body, and can provoke inflammation. The omega-3 fats are less likely to cause inflammation and are considered to be more heart-healthy. In addition to fish, they are found in canola oil and to a lesser extent in walnuts and other nuts. Monounsaturated fats are considered to be very heart-healthy and are not likely to trigger inflammation. Good sources include olive and canola oils, and nuts. Let's learn a little more.

Which Fats?

Okay, so which fats should we choose? What makes a fat heart-healthy? Let's discuss some of the most common fats, including important health information about each.

Olive oil: Olive oil is well-known to be good for your heart and is a very important part of the Mediterranean diet. It is rich in monounsaturated fats, especially oleic acid (so named because it comes from olives). DASH diet studies have shown improvements in blood pressure by replacing empty carbs with olive or canola oil. Olive oil consumption is associated with other benefits, including less inflammation and lower rates of some kinds of cancer.

Fish oils: The omega-3 fish oils, especially DHA (docosahexaenoic acid) and EPA (eicosapentaenoic acid), are known to be very protective for the heart and for the brain. Yes, fish can be considered to be brain food. Studies of the Inuit people in Greenland, who consume high levels of fats, especially from seafood, have shown that they have very low rates of heart attacks. This initially puzzled scientists, until they realized how beneficial these omega-3 fatty acids could be. Especially good plant-food sources of the omega-3 ALA (alpha-linoleic acid), an essential fat, are soy oil, walnuts, peanut oil, flax, and canola oil. Our bodies can turn ALA into the more beneficial DHA but are relatively inefficient at it, so we benefit more from fish oils. In addition to heart and brain health, these omega-3s help reduce inflammation. You probably know someone with rheumatoid arthritis, which is an especially obvious case of inflammation. But there is also low-level inflammation going on throughout your body. Inflammation is associated with initiating and maintaining many diseases, including the formation of plaque in your arteries and the development of type 2 diabetes, Alzheimer's disease, and many types of cancer. Omega-3s will help reduce your levels of inflammation. One marker that your diet is helping to reduce inflammation is a significant decline in triglyceride levels. C-reactive protein (CRP) is another marker that can identify lower levels of inflammation, but it is not routinely tested.

What about fish oil supplements?

If you are taking fish oil supplements, the most recent studies have shown that they do not appear to help reduce the risk of heart disease or heart attacks. This discrepancy with previous recommendations is believed to be because people are now aggressively treated to manage heart disease, leaving little room for improvement from supplements. Long-term data still show a strong heart-protective benefit from consuming fish rich in omega-3 fats, as is recommended in the Mediterranean diet, and supplements have been shown to help lower triglycerides.

Flaxseed: Although flaxseed contains high levels of the essential omega-3 ALA, I personally am not a fan because of the high oxidative potential of flax oil. As we discussed, oxidation can be the first step in initiating some kinds of cancer (which is why antioxidants are so very important in your diet). Flax oil (also known as linseed oil) is highly susceptible to oxidation, which, in the realm of oils, means it goes rancid quickly. This is not something you want happening in your foods or in your body. (If you do decide to use flax oil or seeds, keep them refrigerated to avoid rancidity, and don't grind seeds until just before use.) Fats that oxidize easily will "consume" antioxidants in your body, an undesirable state of affairs. The people who promote it counter that flaxseeds also contain lignans, which have antioxidant potential. However, during digestion, the oil and the lignans are separated and each go their own way. There is no indication that flax oil is protected from oxidation once it is in your body. It isn't even protected in the seeds.

Furthermore, ALA is very poorly converted to DHA in the body, and DHA and EPA are the omega-3 fats that are truly beneficial for heart health. When evaluating the health benefits of foods, I believe that the most powerful evidence is how it affects health over the long term. There is no long-term evidence of people eating flaxseeds throughout history, although flax was widely grown for making linen. Generally, foods that can be harmful to health are not part of traditional cultural eating habits.

The flax lignans are phytoestrogens (plant estrogens) that have mild estrogenic activity in the human body. Anyone with a history of ER+ breast cancer, or any gynecological cancer, might want to avoid flax.[1]

Monounsaturated fats (MUFA) are a key part of the Mediterranean diet. Nuts, olives, avocados, olive oil, sesame oil, and canola oil are all great sources of heart-healthy MUFA, and they are less suscep-

What Kinds of Fats Should You Definitely Avoid or Limit?

Saturated and trans fats. Saturated fats are the building blocks for making cholesterol in the body. (Even trendy coconut oil, so heavily promoted and propped up by industry-paid research, can cause increased cholesterol.) Trans fats have been identified as bad actors when it comes to heart disease. They are polyunsaturated fats (PUFA) that have been converted into a more saturated form and, unfortunately, have been found to act as if they were SFA. Up until a few years ago, they were in common use to make processed foods that needed to be crispy or crunchy. But now they have been removed from most foods. Unfortunately, in many cases, the foods were reformulated, trans fats having been replaced with saturated fats from palm oil or coconut oil. Those fats are just as bad. The easy way to avoid these fats is to reduce your intake of processed foods. When you make your own meals, you control what goes into it.

Saturated fats also trigger inflammation by activating inflammatory cells.[2] Inflammation, as we have discussed, is associated with increased risk for type 2 diabetes, heart disease, and high blood pressure as well as rheumatoid arthritis, suppressed immune function, and accelerated aging.

tible to oxidation and rancidity than PUFA. Back in the '70s, people were directed toward corn oil and soy oil for heart health. However, they are high in potentially inflammation-increasing omega-6 PUFA and are more susceptible to oxidation. Olive oil has been shown to benefit heart health, and so is a much better choice than the soy and corn oils that were recommended for decades.

Omega-3 fatty acids: The key fish oils are long-chain PUFA fats with two or more double bonds. Omega-3s have one of these double bonds three carbon atoms in from the end of the chain, which is why it is called omega-3. These fats include ALA and the particularly beneficial DHA and EPA. Omega-3 fats are beneficial for lowering triglycerides, as well as for mental health, brain health, and vision.

Essential fatty acids include the omega-6 fatty acid linoleic acid (LA) and the omega-3 fatty acid ALA. (An essential fat is one that is essential for health but that your body cannot make on its own, so it must be derived from foods. They should not be confused with essential oils, which are the essences of certain plants.) You want to have more of the anti-inflammatory omega-3 fats in your diet and less of the omega-6 fats. Arachidonic acid (AA) is an omega-6 PUFA made in your body from LA, which can be either beneficial or harmful, depending on the level in your system. Although AA helps to control inflammation at low levels, excessive amounts can trigger rampant inflammation, as can LA, although it is an essential fatty acid. Dietary DHA and EPA fish oils are long-chain omega-3 PUFA that are associated with lower total cholesterol, lower triglycerides, and reduced blood clotting risk. In the United States, dietary omega-6 PUFA come primarily from corn oil and soybean oil. These are precisely the oils that were recommended since the early 1970s as replacements for solid fats like butter. They became widely used in our homes and in the preparation of processed foods. They are relatively neutral tasting and inexpensive, so they have been used extensively. If you consume a high ratio of omega-6 to omega-3 fats, you may have more inflammation. Most experts recommend a ratio of 4:1 to 1:1. The typical American diet is in excess of 10:1, which may be a factor in the current epidemics of chronic disease related to inflammation.

All in all, the Med-DASH message is to consume more MUFA, more omega-3s from fish, and fewer fats with omega-6 PUFA to reduce inflammatory activity. We are no longer obsessing about limiting all fats.

Protein

If you don't get enough protein, you will lose muscle and your metabolism will slow. Today people are encouraged to get more protein, especially women, the elderly, and people trying to lose weight. The more muscle you have, the faster your metabolic rate, and the healthier you will be. Loss of muscle is one of the key causes of frailty and disability in the aged.

The best-quality protein for sustaining growth and maintaining muscle is egg albumin, closely followed by milk whey protein, beef, and casein (the chief protein in cow's milk). The quality is primarily due to the mix of essential amino acids in these animal proteins but is also impacted by digestibility. However, it is possible to be perfectly well nourished from eating a vegetarian or vegan diet. At one time it was thought that vegetarians had to have "complementary" proteins at each meal in order to have the right amino acid mix to allow for rebuilding and repair of muscle and other tissues. For example, some plant-based foods that are complementary are rice and beans, peanut butter and wheat bread, and corn and beans. In each of these combinations, one food fills in some of the amino acid inadequacies of the other. Together, they make foods that behave just the same as the complete proteins. We no longer believe that it is critical for adults to have complementary proteins at the same meal. Adults have a large mix (a "pool") of free amino acids floating around in the bloodstream, so there are adequate amounts of the right amino acids to fill in for any deficiencies in an individual food to have normal protein metabolism for body maintenance and repair and keeping (or building) strong muscles. Children, however, can benefit from food combining to have the complementary proteins at their meals.

Both vegetarians and omnivores (people who eat meat and plant foods) will get sufficient protein on the Med-DASH plan. You will easily satisfy your protein needs with both plant foods and animal foods. The best sources for animal proteins, in terms of their overall health profile, include eggs, low-fat and nonfat dairy, lean beef and pork, skinless chicken (especially white meat), and fish and other seafood. Lamb is high in cholesterol and saturated fats, so that is an occasional food, if you choose. It is a common part of the Mediterranean diet, so we have included a few recipes for lamb.

Carbs

In many fad diets, "carbs" is considered a dirty word. Certainly, processed grains and added sugars are not essential to anyone's diet and are basically empty calories which most of us don't need.

In the original DASH diet research, carbs were used to provide enough calories so that people did not lose weight during the study period. If the participants had lost weight, it would have made it difficult to evaluate whether the diet pattern or weight loss was the beneficial factor for lowering blood pressure. Subsequent DASH diet research has shown that replacing empty carbs with either protein-rich foods or higher levels of MUFA-rich fats actually gave significantly improved blood-pressure-lowering benefits compared with the higher-carb plan and, as a side benefit, helped to lower triglycerides.

The carbs that break down to simple sugars during digestion are sugar and starch. The primary food sugars (disaccharides) include sucrose (table sugar), lactose (the sugar in milk), and maltose, which break down to glucose and fructose (sucrose), glucose and galactose (lactose), and two glucose molecules (maltose). Honey is a combination of fructose and glucose, a little higher in fructose than glucose. It is not considered to be any healthier than regular table sugar and is actually similar in content to high-fructose corn syrup (HFCS).

We don't need to debate the health aspects of HFCS, because when you are choosing mostly unprocessed foods, it rarely makes its way onto your table. You will be supported here in avoiding most food additives, including artificial sweeteners. This is one of the biggest changes over the past few years. Consumers are demanding foods without these sweeteners. (We are also not going to debate artificial sweeteners here. You will be supported with whatever decision is important for you.) That doesn't mean that we should jump into beverages with lots of added sugars. Later in the book there are some suggestions for ways to add a little sweetness and flavor to water without artificial sweeteners or teaspoons of sugar.

During absorption of your digested foods, glucose can be converted to fructose, and vice versa. Both glucose and fructose end up in your bloodstream, but glucose is the sugar that gets measured when people have diabetes. Insulin is required for glucose to be taken up by muscle tissue, whereas fructose does not need insulin to be metabolized. Fructose is more likely to be used by the liver to make triglycerides either for storage (which can result in fatty liver) or for pumping out into the bloodstream.

Let's not forget the most important carbohydrate class, and the one most lacking in the typi-

Fear of Fructose?

Does the fructose in fruit make it a bad choice? Not at all. Remember all those antioxidants? And fiber? Whole fruit with intact fiber (i.e., not pulverized in a blender) sends its sugar into your bloodstream slowly, so it doesn't give you a sugar rush. Most fruits actually have approximately equal amounts of glucose and fructose. Based on the total weight of the fruit, the sugar contents are quite low, because fruits are mostly water. For example, 1 ounce (28 g) of raspberries (about 15 berries) has 15 calories, 1 gram of sugar, and 2 grams of fiber. Add a small handful of nuts to further slow the absorption of this snack, and it will leave you feeling full for a long time.

cal American diet: fiber. Fiber-rich foods tend to be very filling and tend to be associated with lots of other nutrients. Since fiber only comes from plant foods, fiber-rich foods also tend to be great sources of antioxidants and vitamins and minerals. In my undergraduate classes, we were taught that fiber doesn't provide any calories. However, they actually provide about 10 percent of our calories as the result of breakdown by bacterial fermentation in the colon. We can absorb the gases formed from this fermentation, and some are quite beneficial for keeping us healthy and lean.

The two main types of fiber are soluble and insoluble, although in many scientific reports, two additional classifications are now being used: viscous (usually soluble fiber) and fermentable. Viscous means the fiber thickens the digested food passing through the intestinal tract, which would be beneficial for slowing absorption of glucose. Good examples of viscous fibers are Metamucil (psyllium fiber), pectin (a thickening agent for jams and jellies), and fructooligosaccharides in fruit. Fermentable fibers would include the fiber in beans (gas formers!), oats and barley (beta-glucan), and fruits and vegetables. On the other hand, wheat bran and cellulose are mostly unfermentable, and help with keeping you regular. Having a diet rich in fruits and vegetables is associated with lowering the undesirable LDL cholesterol, while leaving the protective HDL cholesterol high. High-fiber diets are also associated with lower markers of inflammation (CRP) and improved blood pressure. Diets rich in soluble fiber are associated with a lower risk of developing type 2 diabetes. And most diabetes professionals also recommend lots of soluble fiber to help manage blood sugar levels. Fiber from whole (unprocessed) foods is associated with lower weight and improved satiety from meals.[3]

Who doesn't love fresh fruits? They are real treasures in terms of having plenty of beneficial fiber for promoting a healthy gut. My favorites of all are the...Well, okay. Maybe they are all my favorites, depending on the time of year. Tangerines in winter. Berries are available all year round, and I love them on my cereal. But in the summer, I love to make multi-berry pies with strawberries, raspberries, and blueberries. So rich in antioxidants (which give them their blue-purple color), and such a fun treat. If you are limiting processed foods in your diet, you can still have room for these indulgences. In summer I also am addicted to stone fruits, including cherries, plums, nectarines, and peaches. As autumn rolls around, I love to make apple pies or crisps. (I love pies in general; to my friends I am the Queen of Pies.) And almost all year round, we can have melons or bananas at breakfast. Pineapples, papayas, and super-ripe mangoes can make a great dessert or even a salsa for topping mild-flavored fish.

Vegetables of all kinds are other terrific sources of both soluble and insoluble fiber. I personally don't care for hot cereals, but most people do, and you probably know that oatmeal and barley are rich in soluble fiber that helps lower cholesterol and can be very filling. I do love cold cereals, such as the whole-wheat or bran cereals, which help to keep you regular. When they are topped with milk, you get a dairy serving; adding berries or bananas brings in fruit and additional fiber. If you eat breakfast at work, you can bring a cup of fruit yogurt and mix dry cereal into it. There are so many ways to add delicious fiber-rich foods into your diet.

The very important point of the Med-DASH program is that you are eating mostly unprocessed or minimally processed foods, such as yogurt, cheeses, milk, and frozen vegetables and fruits. You could also add fresh (or frozen) meat, poultry, and seafood to that list of minimally processed foods. If you choose to eat more unprocessed foods, with few or no additives, it is very easy to follow the Med-DASH eating plan.

CHAPTER 7

Real Food, Real Easy

The Med-DASH eating plan may seem like it is going to be a challenge. Most Americans don't eat lots of fruits and vegetables. We don't consume enough dairy, and we might miss out on having enough fish in our diet. We need to make this plan fit into our real lives.

Stock Up to Make It Easy!

In order to make it easy to stay on track with the Med-DASH plan, you want to have the right foods on hand. Even if you don't cook, you will find that it is so easy to make healthful meals and snacks when you can go to the fridge and find fresh fruits and veggies, a carton of yogurt, hard-boiled eggs, some sliced cheese, nuts, sliced meats, tuna salad, whole-wheat bread, lettuce...Even if you went looking for chocolate, perhaps some strawberries will call out to you instead. You have the urge for a snack, you open the fridge, and there is a fresh plum and a cup of yogurt. How much more appetizing than some junk snack that won't truly satisfy your hunger.

The heart of the Med-DASH plan is plant-based foods: fruits, vegetables, olive oil, beans, nuts, seeds, and mostly whole grains, when you do have grains. Your diet automatically becomes high-fiber and full of antioxidants, vitamins, and minerals. Fortunately, if you consume dairy, meats, poultry, seafood, or beans, they are also rich in vitamins and minerals and high-quality protein. This is a super-nutritious food plan based mostly on whole foods, and is very easy to follow. Not just a few super-foods, but a complete super–diet plan based on great foods.

Life has become very confusing when it comes to buying groceries. Do you want organic, GMO-free? How about locally grown with sustainable agriculture? I am not going to preach to you. Costs and your personal health concerns can guide your choices. But we don't need to reject foods that have so many health benefits.

I love farmers' markets. I much prefer to buy food from individual growers. They often have the tastiest foods because the produce isn't grown with the sole objective of being able

Organic? Or Not?

Organic foods are great, but not essential for good health. Your budget and your preferences can guide your choices. But please don't let a fear of trace amounts of pesticides deter you from eating fruits and vegetables. While there are rankings of produce, claiming that some are excessively high in pesticides, these are often the foods with the highest health quotient in terms of fiber, vitamins, minerals, and antioxidants. It is your choice whether to buy organic foods or not; just please don't reject fruits and vegetables because of fears about how they were grown. Of course with non-organic foods, you can wash them very well or peel them to limit your exposure to pesticides.

to withstand long-distance transportation. They are grown for flavor! If you are up for it, grow your own. Home gardens produce the tastiest tomatoes, the most tender broccoli. What is the point of eating a tomato if it is mealy and tasteless? (If I can't get to the farmers' market and don't have ripe tomatoes in my garden, I have discovered that heirloom tomatoes in season or grape tomatoes from the grocery store are flavorful and lovely.) The freshest sweet corn is the best tasting. Peaches from smaller farms are so much more delicious. In most areas of the country, you can find locally grown and raised foods, including beef and poultry, dairy, eggs, and seasonal fruits and vegetables. Depending on your budget, it is great to support local growers and to feel a little more connected to the people who produce your food. You and your family are more likely to eat fruits and vegetables when they are super-tasty, organic or not.

What to Choose

Oils

Key MUFA-rich oils include olive and canola. They are less susceptible to rancidity than PUFA oils, but can still become oxidized. You can slow this down dramatically by storing them in the refrigerator, where the cooler temperatures slow oxidation. Even though it is not as economical, I buy smaller bottles of oil to minimize the amount of time I store the opened bottles (and since rancid oil needs to be tossed out, perhaps it *is* more economical to buy oil in smaller quantities). Light will also speed oxidation of fats, so if not in the refrigerator, a dark, cool cupboard is the best place to store oil. This is especially true for olive oil: Since it will partially solidify in the refrigerator, I store it in the coolest, dark spot in my kitchen instead, and buy only small bottles.

Avoiding Rancid Oils and Foods

You can easily smell the difference between fresh and rancid oils. Buy a new bottle and compare it with an older bottle that hasn't been stored in the fridge. Now remember that odor and use it to judge whether your food is fresh. It isn't just the oil in a bottle that can go rancid. Whole grains, including oatmeal, cereals, and flour, can go bad, as can nuts and seeds, some dried beans, crackers, boxed bread crumbs, and chips. And always store natural (additive-free) peanut butter or other nut butters in the refrigerator.

Beans, Nuts, and Seeds

Nuts and seeds should be refrigerated or kept in the freezer to stay fresh because they too can become rancid. Yes, they are high in fat. But surprise! They are super-nutritious and associated with lower cholesterol and reduced risk of heart attacks. Most nuts are rich in MUFA, as well as fiber, potassium, selenium, and other important minerals, and provide key benefits to both the DASH and Mediterranean diets. They may be particularly advantageous to help reduce the risk of type 2 diabetes, and are anti-inflammatory. Beans, of course, are very high in fiber, which may be protective in terms of supporting a good balance of bacteria in the gut. They are excellent sources of protein, especially for people trying to limit their intake of animal foods.

Lean Meats and Poultry

Beef and pork are much leaner today than they were twenty-five years ago. We do, however, want to limit our intake of red meat to two or three times per week. Newer information about the digestive end products of meat show that by-products can be formed that can increase your risk of heart disease. One such end product is trimethylamine (TMA), which can be converted to trimethylamine N-oxide (TMAO) in the liver. TMAO is associated with higher risk for CVD mortality and may increase the tendency of cholesterol to form plaques in arteries. The process of making TMAO seems to be related to an unhealthy balance of bacteria in your gut. The high amount of plant foods in the Med-DASH plan helps to nourish good bacteria and can minimize production of TMAO and the negative effects of including meat in your diet.

The best choices for beef and pork are cuts that have the words "loin," "chop," "chuck," or "round" in their names. These meats are naturally low in saturated fats and calories. You do not need to go super-low fat with beef, since you'll likely end up with tasteless, dry meat that no one will eat. Appendix A provides a listing of beef fat content for different cuts. Pork can also be a great choice. It tends to be raised to be much leaner than it was twenty-five years ago. For this reason, you really want to avoid overcooking pork, which will leave the meat dry and tough. You will find information on the nutrition content of pork in Appendix B. Both beef and pork are great sources of vitamins and minerals. In particular, they are rich in potassium, which appears to be a key part of how the DASH diet helps to lower blood pressure.

Skinless chicken is one of the champions of low-fat meats. Chicken thighs are having a resurgence in popularity, but you might want to make them more of an occasional choice instead of a several times a week option, since they are a little higher in saturated fat. Let your personal taste preference be your guide.

For quick meals and sandwiches (with or without bread), you can buy sliced low-sodium meats at the deli counter. If you would like to have even less processing, though, you can roast your own beef, chicken, or turkey and slice it as thick or thin as you like. The primary health concerns with red meat involve processed meats, so roasting your own is a great way to take charge of your health. Minimize the amount of sausages, bacon, and ham you eat, limiting them to maybe once a month. These foods are fine as an occasional addition to your diet, but take a pass on overconsumption.

Fish and Other Seafood

The very best fish sources of the beneficial fatty acids DHA and EPA are cold-water fatty ocean fish. Great choices include tuna, mackerel, herring, sardines, halibut, salmon, and anchovies. You may not like all of them, but depending on your personal tastes, I'm sure you will find the right ones to enjoy! If you think you don't like fish, perhaps start with species that taste meatier. I learned to eat fish by trying swordfish, which has a meaty flavor and meaty texture. Then it was on to tuna steaks. Same benefit. Now I love fish, especially salmon.

Just because we specifically want to include fish with omega-3 fats doesn't mean other types of fish and seafood aren't good or should be excluded. Lower-fat fish can also be very healthy, as they are lean, protein-rich foods. You have lots of fabulous choices, including tilapia, whitefish, mahimahi, crustaceans like shrimp and lobster, and mollusks like oysters, clams, and scallops.

Fruits and Vegetables

Fruits and vegetables are the core promoters of good health on the Med-DASH plan. They are chock-full of antioxidants, fiber, vitamins, and minerals, and can be super delicious, along with having the side benefit of being very filling. The more different colors you choose, the more health benefits you will reap. You can choose fresh, frozen, or canned (preferably fruits in low-sugar syrup, or low-salt vegetables), if that fits better into your budget. Berries are especially wonderful. Those intense reds and blues are associated with the very powerful antioxidant anthocyanin. Stone fruits (peaches, plums, apricots, cherries, pluots) are very rich in soluble fiber, which slows your absorption of fructose (the fruit sugar) and nourishes good bacteria in your gut; these fruits also contain anthocyanin. Citrus fruits are rich in carotenoids, along with vitamin C. As mentioned earlier, grapefruit can react with some medications in your body, so talk to your physician to see if you should limit grapefruit in your diet (see page 52 for more information). Even though we don't want to overdo them, both sweet potatoes and regular potatoes are rich in potassium and vitamin C. Orange-yellow fruits and vegetables have lots of beta-carotene, along with other powerful antioxidants. Green leafy vegetables also contain lots of the carotenoids, although they are hidden by green chlorophyll. Tomatoes, red bell peppers, and watermelon are rich in lycopene.

Since we want to choose foods that are naturally filling and satisfying, it's best to limit dried fruits like raisins and dried cranberries. Without the water content you'd find in their fresh form, they aren't as filling, so it is easy to overeat them and not become full as fast as you would if you were eating the whole, fresh fruit. It's also better to eat your fruit than drink it, so most often, choose a juicy piece of fruit over fruit juice or fruit smoothies for the most filling way to enjoy fruit. And the most delicious.

Although we know that fiber from whole foods is associated with healthier weight, we have been caught up in a trend that actually reduces fiber from fruits and vegetables: smoothies! Even if your juicer or blender leaves the fiber in, the processing of the smoothies pulverizes the fiber and makes it ineffective. So...enough with the smoothies! You want the fiber. The whole, intact fiber. That is a prime benefit of produce. Eat the fruits and vegetables, don't drink them! It's more filling and helps slow the absorption of sugar, which in turn helps you avoid a sugar rush.

It has been found that the intestinal tracts of vegetarians have a different mix of bacteria than those of non-vegetarians. In general, this mix helps vegetarians stay leaner and avoid becoming overweight, and fiber is one of the key elements of this intestinal good health. It is also a key factor in the health benefits of the DASH diet and the Mediterranean diet.

Dairy

Dairy is important for providing all the blood pressure benefits of the DASH diet. In general, we would like to mostly choose nonfat or reduced-fat dairy. You may think this runs contrary to the "keep the fat in the diet" message of the Med-DASH plan. However, we do want to limit saturated fats, which are associated not only with heart-health concerns but also increased risk for insulin resistance (a precursor to type 2 diabetes), perhaps lower bone density in women, and some kinds of cancer, including prostate cancer. (It should be noted that for men, intake of 2 or more cups of milk per day is associated with an increased risk for prostate cancer, so lower intake may be beneficial.) Calcium and magnesium also reduce the absorption of saturated fats.

Fermented dairy foods, whether Greek yogurt or mozzarella cheese, are very familiar parts of the Mediterranean diet and are easy for most people to digest. The lactose in yogurt or cheese is converted into lactic acid, which is what provides the thickening. The straining process that concentrates Greek yogurt reduces its lactose content even further. Many people even find that their tolerance for dairy improves if they consume more yogurt. In cheese-making, almost all residual lactose gets removed when the liquid whey portion is separated from the solid curds. There are so many important nutrients, such as high-quality protein, calcium, potassium, magnesium, and vitamin D, in dairy foods, so please include them if they agree with you.

Some people, especially as we get older, have blood pressure that is very sensitive to salt. Sodium is added to speed cheese ripening, as well as for flavor and as a preservative. But many types of cheeses are naturally low in sodium, such as Swiss (Emmental), Monterey Jack, mozzarella, ricotta, and cream cheese.

Some people consider nonfat (skim) milk to be a highly processed and unnatural food. Really? For eons, humans have allowed the cream to rise on a container of milk to get the butterfat. I wouldn't really call that "processed." The separation happens all by itself. The question of whether we need to drink skim or reduced-fat milk, however, is a little murkier than originally thought. Several recent studies have shown that drinking whole milk has little effect on blood cholesterol levels.

Eggs

Eggs were once considered to be absolutely forbidden on a heart-healthy diet. Today we are less concerned with dietary cholesterol than we are with the cholesterol the body makes from saturated fats. We normally consume 100 times more saturated fat than cholesterol every day. Our own internal production of cholesterol greatly out-does the amount we eat. The American Heart Association (AHA) advises that eggs can be part of a heart-healthy diet again. To be very specific, the new lifestyle recommendations state that there is no evidence that lowering intake of cholesterol from foods does anything to help to lower LDL ("bad") cholesterol levels.[1]

Eggs are extraordinarily packed with nutrients. Lutein and zea-xanthin are two powerful antioxidants from the carotenoid family. They are very important for eye health, helping to reduce the likelihood of age-related macular degeneration and the development of cataracts. Choline is needed in all body cells and is especially important during fetal development to support brain health. Eggs have the highest-quality protein, which means that it is the most efficiently used form of protein for growth and maintenance of the human body. Additional key vitamins and minerals include vitamin D, iron, selenium, and riboflavin. Most of the nutrients are in the yolk, so don't throw it away!

Eggs make a wonderful breakfast food, because their protein content helps keep you satisfied longer than sugary breakfast cereals or other high-starch foods.

Breads, Pasta, Rice, and Cereal Grains

Grains are all high in starch. In the '90s, starch was called a complex carbohydrate and labeled as slower to digest. In reality, starch is very easy to digest, with the process starting while chewing. It easily is turned into glucose—in fact, it converts 100 percent into glucose. The fiber from whole grains is beneficial for staying regular and may have some anti-oxidant properties. Oats and barley are particularly rich in soluble fiber, which can help lower LDL ("bad") cholesterol and triglyceride levels and slow the absorption of glucose into your bloodstream, as compared with refined grains. Even though we tend to eat sweet corn as if it were a vegetable, in reality, it is a grain, and a whole grain at that. One of the problems with breads is that they are low in water, which makes them relatively non-filling. Rice and pasta will be a little more filling, but are still easily digested. By the weight of food consumed, carbs such as these grains are relatively high in calories, so you may want to limit them, especially if you are trying to get to a healthier weight. I personally like to use vegetables in some of the dishes where I would normally use grains so that I can still enjoy my favorites, but with much lower calories. So there you have it. Grains: healthy if they are mostly whole grains, but best to eat in moderation.

Quinoa

Although some may disagree, quinoa will be classified as a grain in this eating plan. It is mostly starch, with some protein and fat. You may have heard that quinoa is a good source of protein. It is a source of high-quality protein, but it is not high in protein. The nutrient breakdown is similar to that of other grains, at about 80 calories, 15 grams carbohydrates (starch), 3 grams protein, 1 gram fat, and 2 grams fiber per serving (1 ounce dried or about ⅓ cup cooked).

Herbs and Spices

Throughout history, herbs and spices have been used to increase the flavor of foods. Who knew that they also had important health effects? One interesting point is that many spices have antibacterial properties. Those hot, spicy flavorings, which are used in traditional dishes in tropical areas, have mild preservative properties. Spices and herbs are also rich in antioxidants and other bioactive chemicals. Whether it is turmeric for anti-inflammatory properties, or cinnamon for lowering blood sugar, or cancer protection by garlic, there are a host of health-promoting benefits of herbs and spices. The Mediterranean recipes in this book will introduce you to a new world of flavors by incorporating spice palettes from all around the Mediterranean region.

Chocolate

Chocolate is super-rich in antioxidant polyphenols. Studies in several countries have shown that people who have a cup of hot chocolate daily are less likely to have issues with heart disease and blood pressure. Observational studies of people all over the world, including in the United States, Sweden, Holland, the Kuna Indians in Panama, and elsewhere, have shown cardioprotective benefits for people who have moderate chocolate intake. Polyphenol-rich chocolate has been shown to lower blood pressure, improve vascular function, have a vasodilatory effect, reduce oxidative stress, increase mitochondrial function (associated with the capacity to burn off excess energy), reduce platelet stickiness (associated with blood clots), and improve the ability to respond to insulin and metabolize glucose properly.[2] Choose mostly really good dark chocolate, in smallish portions, and enjoy!

Hot Chocolate (or Cocoa)

It's simple to make your own hot chocolate for a morning dairy infusion. In a mug, stir or whisk together 1 cup hot milk, 1 tablespoon unsweetened cocoa powder, and 1 teaspoon sugar (or artificial sweetener if you choose) until well combined.

CHAPTER 8

The Super-Simple Overview: Med-DASH Rules

In this chapter, I will pare down all the guidelines to give you a super-simple overview of what the Med-DASH plan looks like.

Color on your plate.

The more color on your plate, the healthier the meal. The color comes from fruits and vegetables. In general, an easy way to avoid overeating is to have lots of bulky, filling (but not high in starch) vegetables with each meal. Whole fruits will also give you a payoff and keep you full. These foods can play a useful role in the Med-DASH plan for reducing calorie intake without losing any of the satisfaction in your meals. There is no law against having three or more servings of vegetables in a meal. Fiber keeps you feeling full longer, and a colorful meal means lots of antioxidants to help reduce inflammation.

Veggies for Your Spaghetti

I love spaghetti. One of my favorite tricks for cutting down on empty carbs from pasta while still enjoying all the flavor of my homemade spaghetti sauce is to serve it on vegetables instead of pasta for the base. If you can put tomato-based sauces on fish or chicken, why not on vegetables? Have the sauce on broccoli or green beans. Still want the look of pasta? Of course, spiralized zucchini or other squash "noodles" make it so easy to enjoy, while not overdoing what you eat.

Have 3 meals and 2 or 3 snacks every day.

Deprivation does not lead to lasting weight loss. If you are hungry, you should eat. Quench your hunger when it is easier to control. A better strategy is to eat planned meals and snacks on a regular basis throughout your day. But this is not grazing, which isn't a great idea. How do you know when you have grazed enough? Most people don't. Plan your meals and snacks ahead of time so you aren't caught off guard when you're hungry and find yourself eating foods that aren't that healthy.

Add lean, protein-rich foods to satisfy your hunger and keep you from being hungry again an hour later.

Protein foods take longer to digest and be absorbed. The energy (and some glucose produced from the protein amino acids) from protein-rich foods will be entering your bloodstream about the time the carbs are leaving, meaning no sugar crash when you have mixed meals and snacks.

Use dairy to help quench hunger.

Milk is a mixed meal all by itself, since it naturally contains some carbs, a healthy dose of protein, and a little bit of fat. Pair it with something fiber-rich for balance. With milk, whole-grain cereal, and some fruit, you have a quick balanced breakfast, and you are on your way.

Add fresh fruits to satisfy your sweet tooth the healthy way.

If you are craving a sweet snack or a sweet end to your meal, fruits are a great way to satisfy. If you have them on hand, it will be easy to stay on track with your plan.

Nuts and seeds make fun snacks that love your heart.

Surprisingly, nuts can help you lose weight. They are great sources of heart-healthy fats, pack in protein and fiber, and are rich in vitamins and minerals. There is no need to avoid these great, satisfying snacks.

Watch your waistline shrink.

A smaller waist is the outward sign of better metabolic health. By cutting down on blood sugar surges, you won't force your body to plump up your abdominal fat cells with glucose that then gets turned into more fat. Avoid overtaxing your body with lots of simple carbs (and yes, starch is a simple, very quickly digested carb).

PART 2

Customized Meal Plans Just for You!

In the next two chapters, you will find examples of various ways to put the Med-DASH diet plan together. These are suggestions. Please customize the meal plans for your own tastes and preferences. The jump-start program in the next chapter will help you relearn how to eat. It will teach you how to create satisfying meals and snacks, and balance foods to satisfy hunger and avoid cravings. In the jump-start program do not skip any meals or snacks. You do not want to let your hunger get out of control. In the full plan, the afternoon snack is optional, according to your hunger level. This is also a very important foundation of the full Med-DASH plan, and the jump-start program teaches you how to accomplish this. You will get all the benefits of the full plan, but intensified.

Welcome to the Med-DASH program.

CHAPTER 9

Optional Jump-Start and Relearning How to Eat

A key feature of this book is to help you learn a way of eating that makes it easy to reach and maintain a healthy weight and take care of your health at the same time. With the current epidemics of obesity, heart disease, and type 2 diabetes, it's clear that too many of us are doing something wrong.

One of the worst nutrition guidelines ever was the recommendation in the 1992 Food Guide Pyramid that people should eat as many as eleven or twelve servings of grains every day. OMG! Who, outside of marathon runners, could burn up that much carb energy? These recommendations came out exactly as everyone was becoming more sedentary than ever before. (Even if you go to the gym every day, research suggests that it barely makes up for having a sedentary job where you sit all day.[1]) These guidelines were a recipe for disaster, and the present-day epidemics of obesity, heart disease, and diabetes are the result.

When those recommendations were combined with guidance to cut way back on fat and to minimize protein intake, you got meals that were not satisfying and did not quench hunger. Without sufficient protein, people who lost weight also dramatically reduced their metabolic rate, making it virtually impossible to maintain that weight loss.

You are going to re-train yourself to eat in a way that is satisfying and quenches hunger for more than 30 minutes. This jump-start plan lasts from one to two weeks, and completing the jump-start will make it much easier to adopt the full plan. You decide when you are ready to move on to the full Med-DASH eating program. During your jump-start, you will learn to make veggies the center of your plate and protein the satisfying accompaniment. You will avoid starchy and sugary carbs, so you won't have sugar crashes that lead to cravings and all-day grazing.

It is important to focus on "foods to include" instead of what to avoid. In the one to two weeks of the jump-start, you are going to focus on including lots of nonstarchy vegetables; lean meats, fish, or poultry (for nonvegetarians); beans, nuts, and seeds; low-fat or nonfat fermented dairy foods; and heart-healthy fats. This array is the foundation of healthy eating advice and of a truly sound lifelong eating style. The advantage of this jump-start plan is that it helps you learn how to eat in a satisfying way that is filling, while not causing blood sugar highs and lows that can lead to overeating. You will learn to naturally moderate how much you eat.

During this one- to two-week jump-start plan, you are going to avoid carbs: That means fruits, starchy veggies, and grains

Feeding Your Family

You can still make meals for your whole family. Just don't add everything to your plate. Skip the bread. Replace potatoes and pasta with veggies. Make your salad bigger than the rest of the family's. And they still get to eat the way they like. So easy!

are out. But just for one to two weeks. This is a short-term quick fix to maximize your results. And this part is absolutely optional. That said, people do find that this re-training helps them forge a path that is naturally sustainable. And they love the weight loss, especially around the waist.

What We Choose

Protein-rich foods

Lean meats, fish, poultry
Fermented (preferably) reduced-fat dairy foods: cheese, yogurt
Eggs
Beans and peas: These are great protein options for vegetarians. Although they do contain a fair amount of starch, they are also fiber-rich, which slows down how quickly your body digests and absorbs them, so there is little concern for them causing you to have a glucose crash from the starch.

Nonstarchy veggies

This includes almost all vegetables, except, for example, potatoes, yams or sweet potatoes, beets, and parsnips. Sweet corn is a grain, even though we tend to think of it as a vegetable. We are skipping grains during the jump-start.

Heart-healthy fats

Olive, peanut, and canola oils
Nuts and seeds (also good protein sources), including peanuts and peanut butter
Avocados

On Hold?

During this optional jump-start, we are putting a few of the key Med-DASH foods on hold. But just for a week or two. Fruit and whole grains are very healthy, so don't worry, they come right back in after the jump-start. Starchy and sugary vegetables like potatoes, sweet potatoes, parsnips, and beets are foods you want to avoid at this point. All grains are off the table, including wheat, corn, oats, and quinoa. For dairy, we are just going to have small amounts of milk, such as what you'd add to coffee. Yogurt and cheeses are absolutely fine during the jump-start. At this point you are just establishing a new foundation based on protein-rich foods, high-fiber, low-starch, and low-sugar foods; and heart-healthy fats.

How Many Servings?

I like to provide serving size guidance in terms of appetite size: smaller, moderate, or larger. Focusing on calories or being overly rigid doesn't help you learn how to eat in a way that is pleasant or sustainable. I want you to figure out how much to eat based on what is satisfying for you. Without worrying about calories, you still can lose weight. It happens because you are choosing foods that are bulky and filling (fruits and veggies) as well as satisfying (protein and fats). You want to focus on getting a variety of different food types, which will bring you the right mix of nutrients to improve your health. And as you change your eating habits, your hunger level decreases, so you will be satisfied with smaller servings.

The (Optional) Jump-Start Program for Med-DASH

Daily Servings

	Smaller Appetite	Moderate Appetite	Larger Appetite
Nonstarchy vegetables ½ cup cooked, 1 cup raw, 4–6 ounces juice	Unlimited, minimum of 5		
Dairy 1–2 ounces milk in coffee, 4–6 ounces yogurt, 1 ounce cheese	2	2–3	2–4
Nuts, beans, seeds ¼ cup nuts, seeds, nut butter, ½ cup beans	1	1–2	1–2
Lean meat, fish, poultry, eggs	5–6 ounces, cooked	6–8 ounces, cooked	8–11 ounces, cooked
Fats	1–2	2–3	2–4

Table 5. *Detailed serving size descriptions are shown on the tracking form on page 116.*

What do you learn from the jump-start?

- To fill your plate with colorful vegetables and balance them with lean meats, fish, and poultry or other protein-rich foods such as beans.
- To add dairy to your day by choosing milk, cheese, or yogurt.
- That your hunger is easy to manage without the blood sugar highs and lows.

In all the measures for the meal plans and serving sizes, fluid ounces are used for liquids and ounces are used for foods eaten by weight.

And what are the results?

- You will have calmed the inflammation caused by your body's response to your previous intake of excess calories, especially sugars and starches.
- You won't overproduce triglycerides, LDL cholesterol, or the fat-storage hormone insulin.
- You will lose weight and feel great!

What a great start to an eating plan that will improve your health and be easy to follow! It is a new way of eating, one that will become your eating plan for a lifetime.

What does a typical day on the jump-start plan look like?

Breakfast

- Something protein-rich: 1 or 2 eggs, and/or 1 to 2 ounces sliced lean meat, or ½ cup beans or lentils
- Something bulky/filling and rich in vitamin C: Preferably vegetables (or vegetable juice)
- A little milk in your coffee or tea, if desired (sugar is not recommended during the jump-start)

Midmorning snack

- Nuts, 4 to 6 fluid ounces yogurt, or 1 ounce cheese, and raw veggies

Lunch

- Roll-ups: a lettuce wrap, 1 slice (1 ounce) reduced-fat cheese, 2 to 3 ounces lean meat/fish/poultry or beans
- Extra veggies: salads and other raw veggies
- Water with fruit slices (although don't eat the fruit in the jump-start program)
- Light yogurt

Afternoon or before-dinner snack

- Same as morning snacks, plus additional options, such as raw veggies dipped in ¼ cup guacamole, salsa, or hummus

Dinner

- Salad with mixed greens and raw veggies, optional nuts/seeds
- 3 to 5 ounces cooked lean meat, fish, or poultry, or main-dish beans
- 1 or more cups cooked nonstarchy veggies
- Water with fruit slices (don't eat the fruit during the jump-start)

Below is a suggested tracking form for the jump-start plan. You can download larger versions of this form at dashdiet.org/forms

The Med-DASH Food Group Servings Check-Off Form

Food Groups	Monday	Tuesday	Wednesday	Thursday	Friday	Saturday	Sunday
Grains, starches, sweets None in Jump Start							
Fruits None in Jump Start							
Vegetables ½ cup cooked vegetables, 1 cup leafy greens, 6 ounces vegetable juice	☐☐☐☐☐☐	☐☐☐☐☐☐	☐☐☐☐☐☐	☐☐☐☐☐☐	☐☐☐☐☐☐	☐☐☐☐☐☐	☐☐☐☐☐☐
Dairy (preferably low-fat) 1–2 fluid ounces skim or low-fat milk in coffee, 6–8 ounces yogurt, 1 ounce cheese, ½ cup cottage cheese	☐☐☐☐	☐☐☐☐	☐☐☐☐	☐☐☐☐	☐☐☐☐	☐☐☐☐	☐☐☐☐
Beans, nuts, seeds ¼ cup beans, nuts, seeds; 2 tablespoons peanut butter	☐☐☐☐	☐☐☐☐	☐☐☐☐	☐☐☐☐	☐☐☐☐	☐☐☐☐	☐☐☐☐
Lean meat, fish, poultry, eggs, soy meat substitutes Each ☐ = 1 ounce (after cooking) 1 egg = 1 ounce, 2 egg whites = 1 ounce	☐☐☐☐☐ ☐☐☐☐☐	☐☐☐☐☐ ☐☐☐☐☐	☐☐☐☐☐ ☐☐☐☐☐	☐☐☐☐☐ ☐☐☐☐☐	☐☐☐☐☐ ☐☐☐☐☐	☐☐☐☐☐ ☐☐☐☐☐	☐☐☐☐☐ ☐☐☐☐☐
Fats, fatty sauces 1 tablespoon salad dressing 1 teaspoon butter, oil	☐☐☐☐☐☐	☐☐☐☐☐☐	☐☐☐☐☐☐	☐☐☐☐☐☐	☐☐☐☐☐☐	☐☐☐☐☐☐	☐☐☐☐☐☐
Water, liquids 8 ounces	☐☐☐☐☐ ☐☐☐☐☐	☐☐☐☐☐ ☐☐☐☐☐	☐☐☐☐☐ ☐☐☐☐☐	☐☐☐☐☐ ☐☐☐☐☐	☐☐☐☐☐ ☐☐☐☐☐	☐☐☐☐☐ ☐☐☐☐☐	☐☐☐☐☐ ☐☐☐☐☐
Alcohol None in Jump Start							
Exercise (each ☐ = 10 minutes)	☐☐☐☐☐ ☐☐☐☐☐	☐☐☐☐☐ ☐☐☐☐☐	☐☐☐☐☐ ☐☐☐☐☐	☐☐☐☐☐ ☐☐☐☐☐	☐☐☐☐☐ ☐☐☐☐☐	☐☐☐☐☐ ☐☐☐☐☐	☐☐☐☐☐ ☐☐☐☐☐

Grains, starches	_____	Vegetables	_____	Dairy	_____	Fats	_____
Fruits	_____	Beans, nuts	_____	Lean meats	_____	Liquids	_____
Alcohol	_____	Exercise	_____				

7 Days of Jump-Start Meal Plan Examples

These meal plans are examples rather than prescriptions. Follow them to the letter, or just use them for models of the kind of meals you want to eat. You will notice that the portion sizes are flexible. You want to learn for yourself how much of these foods you need to eat in order to be satisfied. And that is the goal. Deprivation and starving yourself do not work in developing a sustainable eating pattern and a healthy weight. You will also note that there are no calorie levels or listing of nutrient composition of the meals. You don't eat calories. You don't eat nutrients. You eat foods, delicious, whole foods. This is a much more positive and enjoyable way to approach healthy eating and healthy weight.

(Recipes found in this book are marked with*.)

Day 1

Breakfast

- 1 or 2 eggs, scrambled
- 1 ounce sliced cooked lean meat, poultry, or fish
- 4 to 6 fluid ounces vegetable juice
- Coffee or tea with a little milk, if needed; or water

Midmorning snack

- 1 ounce light cheese
- 8 baby carrots
- Coffee, tea, or water

Lunch

- 4 ounces tuna on a mixed salad with Vinaigrette*
- Sliced cucumbers

- Tomato
- Water with sliced lemon

Afternoon or before-dinner snack

- 4 ounces light yogurt (Greek or regular)

- **Dinner**
- Pollo alla Griglio*
- 1 cup broccoli
- Water with lemon slices

Day 2

Breakfast

- 1 or 2 hard-boiled eggs
- 8 fresh cherry tomatoes, or 4 to 6 fluid ounces vegetable juice

Midmorning snack

- Cucumber slices
- 1 ounce light cheese

Lunch

- 1 or 2 roll-ups: 1 slice light cheese, 2 ounces sliced turkey breast, and 1 slice tomato rolled up in 1 lettuce leaf
- ½ cup Italian Coleslaw*
- Additional raw veggies, if desired
- Water with orange slices

Afternoon or before-dinner snack

- Small handful of nuts
- Baby carrots

Dinner

- 3 ounces roast beef
- Sautéed carrots and onions:
  In a large skillet, heat 2 tablespoons olive oil over medium heat. Add 1 sliced medium onion and sauté for about 5 minutes or until translucent. Add 2 cups sliced carrots and sauté until desired softness, reducing the heat under the pan as needed to avoid burning. Add 1 thin pat of butter at the end. Serve on top of roast beef for additional flavor.
- Mixed salad with Italian Dressing*
- Water with sliced lemon

Day 3

Breakfast

- 2 to 3 ounces lox (smoked salmon) topped with 1 tablespoon cream cheese or a 1-ounce slice Swiss cheese
- Tomato slices
- Onion slices (if desired)
- Coffee or tea with a little milk if needed

Midmorning snack

- 4 ounces light yogurt
- 20 almonds

Lunch

- Cold cooked skinless chicken breast, with a mixed salad and Vinaigrette*
- Additional raw veggies per your preference
- Water with lime slices

Afternoon or before-dinner snack

- 1 ounce light cheese
- Handful of grape or cherry tomatoes

Dinner

- Hamburger (no bun)
- Grilled onions
- Mixed salad
- 1 cup broccoli
- Water with lime

Day 4

Breakfast

- 1 to 2 ounces sliced turkey with 1 slice light Swiss cheese
- 4 to 6 fluid ounces tomato juice
- Coffee or tea with a small amount of milk, if needed

Midmorning snack

- Raw celery and carrots sticks to dip into 2 tablespoons peanut butter

Lunch

- Large mixed salad topped with grilled chicken and 1 ounce pine nuts
- Water with orange slices

Afternoon or before-dinner snack

- Red or orange bell pepper strips to dip into ¼ cup guacamole

Dinner

- 3 to 4 ounces poached salmon
- Steamed asparagus
- Mixed salad with Vinaigrette*
- Water with lemon slices

Day 5

Breakfast

- Quick mini omelet:
  Put a mini pat (about 1 teaspoon) of butter in the bottom of a small microwave-safe dish. Add 1 or 2 eggs and mix well. Microwave on high for 1½ minutes (or less, if you prefer a less firm omelet). Sprinkle with some cheese.
- Cherry tomatoes or diced tomatoes, inside or on top of the omelet
- Coffee or tea with a small amount of milk, if needed

Midmorning snack

- Cucumber slices to dip into 2 ounces hummus

Lunch

- 1 or 2 roll-ups: about 1 ounce sliced provolone cheese and 1 to 2 ounces sliced lean roast beef, rolled up in 1 lettuce leaf.
- Italian Coleslaw*
- Sliced tomato
- Water with lemon

Afternoon or before-dinner snack

- 4 ounces light yogurt
- 10 cashews

Dinner

- ¼ store-bought rotisserie chicken
- 1 cup cooked frozen mixed broccoli, cauliflower, and carrots
- Mixed salad with Vinaigrette*
- Water with orange slices

Note: This is a great meal when you don't have much time, but still want to put a hot meal on the table. While you are at the store picking up the chicken, hit the salad bar to get a mix of lettuces and toppings for your salad.

Day 6

Breakfast

- 1 or 2 hard-boiled eggs
- 1 ounce lox (smoked salmon)
- Tomato and cucumber slices
- Coffee or tea, with milk if needed

Midmorning snack

- 4 ounces light yogurt
- 10 to 15 cashews

Lunch

- Cheeseburger (no bun)
- Side salad with Ranch Dressing*

- Raw veggies
- Water with lemon

Afternoon or before-dinner snack

- 1 ounce light cheese
- 20 walnuts

Dinner

- Sautéed Chicken with Tomatoes over Haricots Verts*
- Mixed side salad with Lemon Vinaigrette*
- Water with lime

Day 7

Breakfast

- 1 hard-boiled egg
- 1 to 2 ounces sliced turkey
- 4 to 6 fluid ounces tomato juice or a vegetable high in vitamin C

Midmorning snack

- 2 ounces hummus
- 8 celery sticks

Lunch

- 1 or 2 roll-ups: 1 slice Swiss cheese and 2 ounces lean roast beef, topped with grated carrots or other raw vegetables, rolled up in a lettuce leaf
- Italian Coleslaw*
- Tomatoes
- Water with orange slices

Afternoon or before-dinner snack

- 4 ounces light cottage cheese
- 10 baby carrots

Dinner

- Moroccan Cauliflower Pizza*
- Large side salad with Dijon Vinaigrette*
- Water with lemon slices

Beverages

Drink mostly unsweetened beverages, including coffee or tea, preferably with your meals or snacks. Caffeine causes your liver to pump out a little sugar, which could increase hunger if you don't have something to eat at the same time. Water is obviously a great choice. If you prefer it to be a little flavored, you can put some lemon, orange, lime, or cucumber slices in it. This is a nice way to satisfy your sweet tooth without provoking cravings. Just don't eat the fruit during this jump-start phase. And no alcohol until you've moved on to the full program. Please see the beverage section on page 132 in chapter 10 for more discussion on beverages.

Eating on the Run

You can translate any of those meals into restaurant or even fast-food meals.

Breakfast

- Choose eggs, lean meats, and sliced veggies (if available)

Lunch

- Order burgers, grilled chicken, or other sandwiches. Skip the bun or bread.
- Have a side salad or have a big salad with protein-rich toppings

Dinner

- Salad
- Meat, fish, poultry, or beans
- Double-veggie side dish
- Leave before dessert!

Snacks

- Yogurt or cheese, nuts, raw veggies, guacamole or hummus with raw veggies

CHAPTER 10

The Full Med-DASH Eating Plan

Now we have arrived! You understand why the Med-DASH plan and many of its components are so healthy. It's time to put the complete Med-DASH eating plan together.

In this chapter, you will find many sample menus to provide you with lots of ideas on how to put the Med-DASH plan together and make it your own. You can follow them exactly or adapt these ideas according to your personal tastes and food preferences.

Specifically, see Table 6 for servings goals for the eating plan.

See Table 7 for examples of what the eating plan looks like, adjusted for various appetite levels (which is an approximation of what would be appropriate for your body size). I don't want to be overly prescriptive. I want you to learn what works for you. Then you will have a sustainable plan. One that you can live with for the long run.

The Med-DASH Eating Plan

Food Group	Servings
Fruits	3–5
Vegetables	4–5
Dairy	2–3
Lean, protein-rich foods: Meats and poultry Eggs Beans	5–9 ounces per day of meat or meat equivalents Up to 7 eggs per week) ½ cup beans = 1 serving
Fats (omega-3 rich)	2 or more 3-ounce portions per week
Nuts and seeds	5 or more 1 ounce servings per week
Fats and oils	6–10 1 tablespoon servings of added fats
Grains	4–6
Added sugar	0–3
Alcohol (4 ounces wine = 1 fruit)	0–2

Table 6. *Typical servings of Med-DASH plans from 1,600 to 2,400 calories.*

Daily Servings for the Med-DASH Plan

	Smaller Appetite	Moderate Appetite	Larger Appetite
Vegetables, nonstarchy	Unlimited, but at least 4	Unlimited, but at least 5	Unlimited, but at least 5
Vegetables, high starch or sugar: potatoes, beets, sweet potatoes	1–2 or less per week	2–3 or less per week	2–3 or less per week

	Smaller Appetite	Moderate Appetite	Larger Appetite
Fruits	3–5	4–5	4–5
Dairy	2–3	2–3	2–3
Nuts, seeds	1	1–2	1–2
Protein-rich foods			
Lean meat, poultry, fish, eggs, limit red meat to 2 or fewer times per week; include fish at least 2 times per week, ½ cup beans or other meat substitutes = about 3 ounces meat	5–6 ounces	6–8 ounces	8–11 ounces
Fats	2–3	3–4	3–4
Whole grains	2–3	2–3	2–4
Wine (4 ounces = 1 fruit serving)	0–1	0–2	0–2
Chocolate (about 1 cubic inch or ½ ounce	If desired, 3–4 times per week		
Refined grains, sugary foods	Rarely, 2–3 times per week		

Table 7. Detailed serving sizes can be found on our tracking form on page 130.

Keeping Track

You're not counting calories, so how do you know if you are following the plan properly? You count servings from the various food groups. Once you get into the habit of paying attention to the foods in your meals, this will become second nature for you. The following form will help you, and you can download more at dashdiet.org/forms.

The Med-DASH Food Group Servings Check-Off Form

Food Groups	Monday	Tuesday	Wednesday	Thursday	Friday	Saturday	Sunday
Grains, starches, sweets 1 slice bread; ⅓ cup cooked pasta, rice; ½ cup cooked cereal, corn, potatoes; ¼ cup dry cereal; ½ English muffin, bun; 2 cups popcorn; 2 small cookies	☐☐☐☐☐☐ ☐☐	☐☐☐☐☐☐ ☐☐	☐☐☐☐☐☐ ☐☐	☐☐☐☐☐☐ ☐☐	☐☐☐☐☐☐ ☐☐	☐☐☐☐☐☐ ☐☐	☐☐☐☐☐☐ ☐☐
Fruits 4 ounces juice, 1 small fruit, ¼ cup dried fruit, ½ cup canned fruit, 1 cup diced raw fruit	☐☐☐☐☐	☐☐☐☐☐	☐☐☐☐☐	☐☐☐☐	☐☐☐☐☐	☐☐☐☐☐	☐☐☐☐☐
Vegetables ½ cup cooked vegetables, 1 cup leafy greens, 6 ounces vegetable juice	☐☐☐☐☐☐	☐☐☐☐☐☐	☐☐☐☐☐☐	☐☐☐☐☐☐	☐☐☐☐☐☐	☐☐☐☐☐☐	☐☐☐☐☐☐
Low-fat dairy 8 ounces skim or low-fat milk, 8 ounces low-fat or fat-free yogurt, 1 ounce reduced-fat cheese, ½ cup fat-free or low-fat cottage cheese	☐☐☐☐	☐☐☐☐	☐☐☐☐	☐☐☐☐	☐☐☐☐	☐☐☐☐	☐☐☐☐
Beans, nuts, seeds ¼ cup beans, nuts, seeds; 2 tablespoons peanut butter	☐☐☐☐☐	☐☐☐☐☐	☐☐☐☐☐	☐☐☐☐☐	☐☐☐☐☐	☐☐☐☐☐	☐☐☐☐☐
Lean meat, fish, poultry, eggs, soy meat substitutes Each ☐ = 1 ounce (after cooking) 1 egg = 1 ounce, 2 egg whites = 1 ounce	☐☐☐☐☐ ☐☐☐☐☐	☐☐☐☐☐ ☐☐☐☐☐	☐☐☐☐☐ ☐☐☐☐☐	☐☐☐☐☐ ☐☐☐☐☐	☐☐☐☐☐ ☐☐☐☐☐	☐☐☐☐☐ ☐☐☐☐☐	☐☐☐☐☐ ☐☐☐☐☐
Fats, fatty sauces 1 tablespoon salad dressing 1 teaspoon butter, oil	☐☐☐☐☐☐	☐☐☐☐☐☐	☐☐☐☐☐☐	☐☐☐☐☐☐	☐☐☐☐☐☐	☐☐☐☐☐☐	☐☐☐☐☐☐
Water, liquids 8 ounces	☐☐☐☐☐ ☐☐☐☐☐	☐☐☐☐☐☐ ☐☐☐☐☐	☐☐☐☐☐ ☐☐☐☐	☐☐☐☐☐ ☐☐☐☐	☐☐☐☐☐ ☐☐☐☐	☐☐☐☐☐☐ ☐☐☐☐☐	☐☐☐☐☐☐ ☐☐☐☐☐
Alcohol 1 ounce liquor, 3 ounces wine, 12 ounces light beer	☐☐	☐☐	☐☐	☐☐	☐☐	☐☐	☐☐
Exercise (each ☐ = 10 minutes)	☐☐☐☐☐ ☐☐☐☐	☐☐☐☐☐ ☐☐☐☐☐	☐☐☐☐☐ ☐☐☐☐☐	☐☐☐☐ ☐☐☐☐	☐☐☐☐ ☐☐☐☐	☐☐☐☐☐ ☐☐☐☐☐	☐☐☐☐☐ ☐☐☐☐☐

____ Grains, starches   ____ Vegetables   ____ Dairy   ____ Fats

____ Fruits   ____ Beans, nuts   ____ Lean meats   ____ Liquids

____ Alcohol   ____ Exercise

What's on your plate in a typical day?

Here is an example. At the end of the chapter, there are fourteen days of sample meal plans.

Breakfast

- Eggs
- Latte
- 4 fluid ounces orange juice
- ½ large banana

Midmorning snack

- 4 ounces strawberries
- 2 ounces nuts (small handful)

Lunch

- Large mixed salad
- Grilled salmon
- Nectarine
- Water with lemon slices

Afternoon or before-dinner snack

- Bell pepper strips dipped in 2 ounces hummus

Dinner

- Mixed side salad
- 3 to 5 ounces roasted chicken breast
- 1 cup broccoli
- 4 fluid ounces red wine
- Water with lemon slices
- 2 ounces raspberries

Beverages

Coffee

Coffee has many health benefits. While it may be under the gun for potentially having a minuscule amount of a cancer-promoting chemical, in real life there appear to be some very important health benefits to coffee. Many studies have shown that people who drink the most coffee are less likely to develop type 2 diabetes. It may reduce your risk of developing Parkinson's disease, liver cancer, and other liver disease. Caffeine may give you a short-term increase in blood pressure, but seems to be heart healthy in general. Coffee is rich in potassium, which is beneficial for improving blood pressure, and most people don't get an adequate amount of potassium in their diet. And coffee is the top source of antioxidants in the typical American diet!

Tea

The health benefits of tea have long been promoted throughout human history. In addition to providing a calming break in your day, tea is another very powerful source of antioxidants. It is associated with better lipid profiles (cholesterol and triglycerides) and reduced risk for heart attack.

Flavored Water or Infused Water

Instead of soda or other sweetened beverages, let's try water with fruit slices. This is such an easy way to get flavor while making the water even more refreshing. Lemon, lime, or orange slices are my favorites. You can also try chunks of melon, such as cantaloupe and watermelon, or cucumber slices. Throw in some herbs, such as fresh cilantro, mint, basil, or rosemary. Add some Tabasco if you like it hot. Another alternative is to make some ice cubes from fresh lemon or orange juice. Drop one or two cubes in your water, and you have the perfect alternative to high-calorie beverages.

Wine and Other Alcohol

Wine is a key part of most meals in the European countries situated around the Mediterranean Sea. Research has shown that people who consume moderate amounts of alcohol live longer than people who do not drink any alcohol. (This does not mean we are encouraging anyone to drink.) Red wine is especially high in antioxidants, and so is grape juice. On this plan, a 3- to 4-ounce glass of wine replaces one serving of fruit. "Moderate" daily intake of alcohol has different definitions depending on the country. By U.S. standards, moderate drinking would be one 4-ounce glass per day for women and two glasses for men, while in some countries, moderate intake is considered two glasses for women and up to three glasses for men.

Milk

Milk is a key component of the DASH diet. The original research showed that the blood-pressure-lowering benefit was not as strong without dairy. Unfortunately, not everyone can tolerate milk sugar, lactose, while some people have a sensitivity to milk proteins. If you can't drink cow's milk, you may be able to substitute goat's milk or a new type of cow's milk called a2. For some people, a2 cow's milk, which has a different form of protein, may be more easily tolerated. Not all stores carry this milk, but you can check a2milk.com to find locations near you. When I was young, I discovered that drinking regular milk caused me severe pain, which I thought was related to a possible ulcer. No ulcer, but I found that when I discontinued drinking milk, I had no more pain. After quite a long time, I started consuming yogurt. After repopulating my gut with beneficial bacteria, I found that I was able to tolerate milk with no subsequent pain. Perhaps you will find that one of these approaches might allow you to include dairy in your meals. Or you may find that yogurt is easier to digest than milk. Most of the lactose in milk

Milk Alternatives

Soy milk has the most comparable nutritional profile to dairy milk. Most brands will have similar amounts of protein, calcium, and potassium as real milk.

Almond milk is mostly water with a few almonds (less than a handful). Depending on the brand, it might or might not have similar calcium or potassium to dairy milk, but no brands have the same amount of protein as real milk.

Coconut milk is high in saturated fats, which can increase cholesterol and raise your risk of developing type 2 diabetes.

Rice milk is low in protein, high in sugars, and low in potassium, but is normally fortified with calcium to make it comparable to milk.

is converted to lactic acid during the fermentation process and is precisely what thickens milk into yogurt and gives it the tang.

Milk substitutes include soy, almond, coconut, and rice milks. It is unknown whether these dairy substitutes provide the exact heart-health benefits as real cow's milk. For milk substitutes, look for brands that contain similar levels of protein, calcium, and potassium as regular milk. If you are just using it in coffee, all options are on the table. Choose what works for you.

Beverages to Avoid or Limit

Fruit juice. Limit juice to a 4- to 6-ounce serving per day. If you've heard people talk about juice belly (particularly in young children), you know what juice can do. Choose whole fruits instead. With all the fiber. Eat most of your fruit, instead of drinking it.

Smoothies. Beware! Yes, smoothies. I know. Everyone thinks they are so healthy. "You can drink much more fruit and/or veggies than you would normally eat." Let's think about why the fruits and veggies are so important. They are our best sources of fiber and antioxidants. And as mentioned earlier, the very act of whipping air into the beverage neutralizes much of the antioxidant potential. Those whirring blades also pulverize the fiber, destroying any advantage that it would provide. Whole fruits and veggies will make you full quicker and will keep you feeling full for a longer period of time. This is such a super trick for moderating your appetite, so you do not want to give it up. Bulky and filling are key strategies for this program. It's so much better to eat yogurt and a banana instead of making them into a smoothie.

Sample Meal Plans for 14 Days

(Recipes found in the book are marked with *.)

Day 1

Breakfast

- 1 ounce (by weight) whole-grain cereal
- 8 fluid ounces milk
- 4 ounces strawberries
- Coffee, tea (could be lattes), or hot chocolate (with little or no sugar added)

Midmorning snack

- Raw carrots
- 2 ounces hummus

Lunch

- 1 or 2 roll-ups: 1 to 2 ounces turkey, 1 ounce cheddar cheese, and sliced tomato rolled up in a lettuce leaf
- Mixed salad with Vinaigrette*
- Plum
- Water with orange slices

Afternoon or before-dinner snack

- 1 ounce mixed nuts
- 4 to 6 ounces light yogurt

Dinner

- 3 to 5 ounces grilled salmon
- Spinach-Arugula Salad with Nectarines and Lemon Dressing*
- Water with lemon slices
- 4 fluid ounces red wine

Day 2

Breakfast

- ⅓ cup cooked oatmeal
- 2 ounces blueberries
- 4 fluid ounces orange juice
- Latte, coffee or tea, or hot chocolate

Breakfast Strategy

The breakfast strategy is that a latte or hot chocolate can easily bring in a dairy serving, or you could substitute a glass of milk or cup of yogurt.

Midmorning snack

- Small handful of almonds
- 6 ounces light yogurt

Lunch

- Cheeseburger (no bun or on a whole-wheat bun)
- 1 cup Italian Coleslaw*
- Water with orange slices
- Small nectarine

Afternoon or before-dinner snack

- Sliced bell pepper strips with Sweet Potato Hummus*

Dinner

- Mixed green salad with Vinaigrette*
- Roast chicken breast:
  Preheat the oven to 400°F. Put skinless chicken breasts in a baking pan, drizzle with 2 tablespoons olive oil, and sprinkle with salt and pepper. Roast for 30 to 40 minutes.
- Roasted carrots, onions, and Brussels sprouts:
  Roast the vegetables in the same pan with the chicken, or line a baking sheet with foil. Cut 1 pound carrots on an angle into 2-inch slices, cut 1 medium onion into half-moons, and cut 1 pound Brussels sprouts in half. Spread the vegetables in an even layer on the pan with the chicken or on the foil-lined pan, drizzle with 1 tablespoon olive oil, and sprinkle with rosemary, thyme, and sage, according to your taste preferences. Roast for 25 minutes, if separate from the chicken.
- 4 fluid ounces red wine
- Flavored water

Day 3

Breakfast

- Small omelet (see page 121)
- Small wedge of cantaloupe
- 6 ounces Greek yogurt
- Coffee, tea, or hot chocolate

Midmorning snack

- 20 cashews
- 1 small apple

Lunch

- Ham and Swiss cheese sandwich:
  2 slices whole-wheat bread, 2 ounces or more lean ham,
  1 ounce Swiss cheese, lettuce and sliced tomato, mustard
  as desired
- Additional slices of tomato or mixed green salad with Citrus
  Vinaigrette*
- 2 small tangerines
- Flavored water

Afternoon or before-dinner snack

- 8 baby carrots dipped in 2 tablespoons natural peanut butter

Dinner

- Roasted Cauliflower Steaks with Chermoula*
- Sautéed halibut
- Mixed green salad with Italian Vinaigrette*
- Flavored water
- 4 fluid ounces red wine

Day 4

Breakfast

- 1 hard-boiled egg
- 4 ounces strawberries

- 20 cashews
- Latte, coffee or tea, or hot chocolate

Midmorning snack

- ½ banana
- 4 ounces Greek yogurt

Lunch

- Cold roast chicken (left over from the previous night; see page 137)
- Italian Coleslaw*
- Sliced small peach (or canned peach in light syrup)

Afternoon or before-dinner snack

- Grape tomatoes and burrata cheese, topped with fresh basil, balsamic vinegar, and 1 teaspoon olive oil

Dinner

- Paella-Style Skillet* (with or without rice; a serving of cooked rice is ⅓ cup, but could be extended by adding more peas)
- Spinach-Arugula Salad with Nectarines and Lemon Dressing*
- Flavored water
- 4 fluid ounces red wine

Day 5

Breakfast

- ¼ cup granola, mixed into 6 fluid ounces Greek yogurt
- ½ banana

- 10 almonds
- Coffee, tea, or hot chocolate

Midmorning snack

- Sliced radishes (or other raw vegetables) and 2 ounces hummus

Lunch (Vegetarian/Vegan)

- Lentil Soup with Sorrel*
- ½ almond butter sandwich made with 1 slice whole-wheat bread topped with 2 tablespoons almond butter
- Small mixed green salad with Lemon-Dill Vinaigrette*
- 1 cup cherries
- Flavored water

Afternoon or before-dinner snack

- Roasted Chickpeas with Herbs and Spices*
- Small plum

Dinner

- Paella-Style Skillet*
- Watermelon Burrata Salad*
- Flavored water
- 4 fluid ounces red wine

Day 6

Breakfast

- Cinnamon raisin bread toast
- ½ banana

- 20 almonds
- Latte, coffee or tea, or hot chocolate

Midmorning snack
- 8 baby carrots dipped in 2 tablespoons natural peanut butter

Lunch
- Tunisian Bean Soup with Poached Egg*
- Small mixed green salad with Vinaigrette*
- 2 small tangerines
- Flavored water

Afternoon or before-dinner snack
- Sweet-and-Spicy Nuts*

Dinner
- Moroccan Cauliflower Pizza*
- Greek Black-Eyed Pea Salad*
- Water with cucumber slices
- 4 fluid ounces red wine

Day 7

Breakfast
- Small spinach omelet
- Sliced cucumbers and tomatoes
- 4 fluid ounces orange juice
- Latte, coffee or tea, or hot chocolate

Midmorning snack

- 6 ounces Greek yogurt
- 20 almonds or cashews

Lunch

- Moroccan Chickpea and Green Bean Salad with Ras el Hanout*
- Small peach
- Flavored water

Afternoon or before-dinner snack

- Sliced bell peppers with ⅓ cup guacamole

Dinner

- Spanish-Style Pan-Roasted Cod* (3 to 5 ounces cooked cod)
- Rice Pilaf with Dill* (⅓ to ⅔ cup)
- Mixed green salad with Citrus Vinaigrette*
- Flavored water
- 4 fluid ounces red wine

Day 8

Breakfast

- Tartine with cream cheese and strawberries:
  This recipe is from *The Everyday DASH Diet Cookbook* by Marla Heller, MS, RD. Toast 1 slice whole-wheat (or other whole-grain) bread, spread with 2 tablespoons whipped reduced-fat cream cheese, and top with slices from 2 large strawberries.
- 2 ounces strawberries (additional)

- 4 fluid ounces orange juice
- Latte, coffee or tea, or hot chocolate

Midmorning snack

- 6 ounces Greek yogurt
- 20 cashews

Lunch

- Cold roast chicken breast (see page 137)
- Greek Potato Salad*
- Plum
- Flavored water

Afternoon or before-dinner snack

- Roasted Chickpeas with Herbs and Spices*

Dinner

- Tortilla Española*
- Salad of mixed frisée and baby butter lettuces, with grape tomatoes and pine nuts, topped with Maltese Sun-Dried Tomato and Mushroom Dressing*
- Apricot and Mint No-Bake Parfait*
- Flavored water
- 4 fluid ounces red wine

Day 9

Breakfast

- Whole-grain cereal
- 4 ounces raspberries

- 1 cup milk
- 4 fluid ounces orange juice or cranberry juice
- Coffee, tea, or hot chocolate

Midmorning snack

- 8 baby carrots dipped in 2 tablespoons natural peanut butter

Lunch

- Red Lentils with Sumac*
- Large mixed salad topped with Lemon-Dill Vinaigrette*
- Small nectarine
- Flavored water

Afternoon or before-dinner snack

- Marinated Olives*

Dinner

- Pan-grilled tilapia, topped with Domatosalata (Sweet-and-Spicy Tomato Sauce)*
- Roasted Vegetable Salad*
- Sliced pear
- Flavored water
- 4 fluid ounces red wine

Day 10

Breakfast

- Small omelet
- 1 slice whole-grain toast

- 4 ounces strawberries
- Latte, coffee or tea, or hot chocolate

Midmorning snack

- Cucumber slices dipped in salsa

Lunch

- 1 or 2 roll-ups: 1 to 2 ounces turkey, 1 ounce cheddar cheese, and sliced tomato rolled up in a lettuce leaf
- Mixed salad with Vinaigrette*
- Small pear
- Flavored water

Afternoon or before-dinner snack

- 4 ounces Greek yogurt
- 20 almonds

Dinner

- Salmon Niçoise Salad with Dijon-Chive Dressing*
- Almond Rice Pudding*
- Flavored water
- 4 fluid ounces red wine

Day 11

Breakfast

- 2 hard-boiled eggs
- ½ banana
- 4 fluid ounces orange juice
- Latte, coffee or tea, or hot chocolate

Midmorning snack

- 6 ounces Greek yogurt mixed with ¼ cup granola

Lunch

- Salmon Niçoise Salad* (left over from the night before)
- Small Granny Smith apple
- Flavored water

Afternoon or before-dinner snack

- Sliced vegetables dipped in ⅓ cup guacamole

Dinner

- Chicken and Chickpea Skillet with Berbere Spice*
- Grain-Free Kale Tabbouleh*
- 4 ounces blueberries mixed with 4 ounces Greek yogurt
- Flavored water
- 4 fluid ounces red wine

Day 12

Breakfast

- Tartine with almond butter and banana:
  Toast 1 slice whole-grain bread, top with almond butter and sliced banana.
- 4 fluid ounces orange juice
- Latte, coffee or tea, or hot chocolate

Midmorning snack

- 6 ounces Greek yogurt mixed with 1 tablespoon sunflower seeds

Lunch

- Cheddar and turkey sandwich:
  2 to 3 ounces sliced turkey, 1 ounce sliced cheddar cheese, lettuce, tomato slices, and mustard on 2 slices light bread
- Italian Coleslaw*
- Small plum
- Flavored water

Afternoon or before-dinner snack

- 10 whole peanuts in the shell

Dinner

- Mixed salad with Vinaigrette*
- Tabil-Spiced Pork Tenderloin with White Beans*
- Mixed cauliflower, broccoli, and carrots, steamed, topped with a small pat of butter, if desired
- 4 ounces fresh pineapple
- Flavored water
- 4 fluid ounces red wine

Day 13

Breakfast

- 2 eggs, scrambled
- Sliced tomatoes
- 4 fluid ounces tangerine-banana juice
- Latte, coffee or tea, or hot chocolate

Midmorning snack

- 6 ounces Greek yogurt
- 20 grapes

Lunch

- Black-Eyed Pea Falafel*
- Small side salad with Citrus Vinaigrette*
- Plum
- Flavored water

Afternoon or before-dinner snack

- Raw vegetables with Garlic-Mint Yogurt Dip*

Dinner

- Mixed green salad with Italian Vinaigrette*
- The Best Spaghetti Sauce*
- Spaghetti, about 3½ inches diameter in your fist for 4 servings
- 8 ounces broccoli
- Sliced fresh peaches
- Flavored water
- 4 fluid ounces red wine

Note: If you want to avoid the pasta, put the sauce on the broccoli, or use zoodles (zucchini noodles).

Day 14

Breakfast

- 1 to 2 slices French toast with strawberries:

In a medium bowl, whisk together ⅔ cup milk, 2 eggs, 1 teaspoon vanilla extract, and 1 teaspoon ground cinnamon. In a large skillet, melt 1 pat of butter over medium heat. Dip 4 slices whole-wheat bread into the milk mixture, coating them well, and place them in the skillet in a single layer. Flip after 3 minutes. Remove from the skillet when the bread has reached your desired level of doneness and set aside on a plate. Repeat with the remaining 4 slices bread. Top with sliced strawberries. Makes 4 servings.

- 4 fluid ounces orange juice
- Latte, coffee or tea, or hot chocolate

Midmorning snack

- Baby carrots dipped in 2 tablespoons natural peanut butter

Lunch

- Couscous Salad*
- Cold rotisserie chicken or roast chicken (see page 137)
- Small Gala apple

Afternoon or before-dinner snack

- Hummus* and raw vegetables

Dinner

- Tabil-Spiced Pork Tenderloin with White Beans*
- Mixed salad with Maltese Sun-Dried Tomato and Mushroom Dressing*
- Diced melon (cantaloupe, honeydew, or your preference)
- Flavored water
- 4 fluid ounces red wine

Entertaining Options

The recipes in chapter 13 give you lots of options for entertaining guests. Here are a couple of suggestions for what to serve at a casual buffet-type party or a more formal sit-down dinner.

Light, Casual Party Fare

Appetizers
- Baked Moroccan-Spiced Chicken Wings*
- Sweet-and-Spicy Nuts*
- Roasted Chickpeas with Herbs and Spices*
- Marinated Olives*
- Domatosalata (Sweet-and-Spicy Tomato Sauce)*
- Raw vegetables
- Hot pita wedges

Dinner
- Watermelon Burrata Salad*
- Tortilla Española*

Dessert
- Ricotta Cheesecake*
- Strawberry–Pomegranate Molasses Sauce* with Greek yogurt

Hearty Meal, Winter Entertaining

First Course
- Spicy Carrot-Orange Soup*

Main Course

- Roasted Vegetable Salad*
- Lamb Tagine*

Dessert

- Almond Rice Pudding*

CHAPTER 11

On Autopilot: Make It Easy and Simple!

Stocking Up

Have you ever thought it was too difficult to eat healthfully? Now is the time to change your mind. The Med-DASH plan can be super-easy to follow. It just depends on having the right foods on hand. This is where you will learn how to set the stage for success. You may have lots of questions about what foods you should choose. Do you need organic? If organic foods fit into your budget, and you prefer them, have at it! What about processed foods? In general, try to choose unprocessed or minimally processed foods. Like locally grown foods? Farmers' markets are the place to go. Or, even better, grow your own! Vegetables are so much tastier when they are homegrown.

Reading Labels

In general, if you are choosing fresh, unprocessed foods, you do not need to worry about food labels.

People who have been trying to lower their blood pressure have heard one thing: Lower sodium intake. However, there can be misconceptions about when sodium in foods is problematic. There is naturally occurring sodium and added sodium. Milk is an example of a whole food that has a fair amount of naturally occurring sodium, but that is not something to avoid, since you get more of the blood-pressure-lowering benefits of DASH when you include milk in the diet than you do without. The added sodium in processed foods is what you want to avoid. Just like with sugars, where we want to limit added sugars. Milk typically has 12 grams of sugar (lactose), but it is not added sugar. Yogurt is even more challenging to understand. The nutrition label reflects the composition of the milk before fermentation. Most of the lactose has actually been converted to lactic acid during that process, so the yogurt's sugar content is thus much lower than it appears to be based on the label. Greek yogurt can have even less residual lactose than regular yogurt.

First, it is important to note that all serving sizes are based on an "as consumed basis." This means that meat, poultry, and fish serving sizes are based on the food's weight after cooking. Cooked grains, like hot cereals, grits, rice, and pasta, are based on the cooked weight. And just to make it more challenging, there are two kinds of ounces. "Fluid ounce" refers to the volume of a liquid, and "ounce" refers to the weight of a solid.

Grains are one area where understanding a serving size usually requires you to read the label. Serving sizes vary dramatically and are very confusing. Flaked cereals will appear to have a larger portion size, while dense cereals (like Grape-Nuts or oatmeal) will look like you are getting a minuscule serving. This is a key point, since many people get totally off track and overdo their calories by thinking that any size bowl is one serving. For example, I had a Sailor who was my patient at a Navy hospital, and came to see me because he couldn't understand why he was gaining weight. It turned out that he was having 1½ cups of Grape-Nuts at breakfast. This is the equivalent of 6 slices of bread. Which brings up another point: We may think of serving size as the portion that we get served. However, in terms of nutrition, serving sizes refer to representative portion sizes that let us compare one food with another. And just to make this really confusing, food labeling requirements call for listing the serving size as the full package if food is sold in a single-serve package. Going back to our cereal example, a prepackaged single-serve cup of Raisin Bran is 2.8 ounces with 280 calories. A standard serving, with 1 ounce of the bran flakes and ½ ounce of raisins, would be 1½ ounces. Not only is the standard serving size different, it is further confounded because of the dried fruit in the cereal. And the Nutrition Facts panel will further try to confuse things by showing that it has 13 grams of sugar. There is little or no added sugar in the bran flakes; most of the sugar comes from the raisins, and fruit is part of our plan. In May 2016, the FDA announced that companies would be required to include new nutrition facts labels on their products. These new labels will identify the quantity of added sugars, to make it easier to understand. (Companies are allowed to take quite a long time to update their labels, however, so as of the printing of this book, we are unsure how long companies will take to fully implement.) The following chart shows a comparison of an old label for a cereal product and a new label for the same cereal. Notice that their serving size of ¾ cup is actually 2 servings of cereal (based on carb grams and calories) for the purposes of tracking your intake. I am continuing to use the serving sizes from the original DASH study, which are typically used in all research on diets. These sizes

SIDE-BY-SIDE COMPARISON

Original Label

Nutrition Facts

Serving Size 2/3 cup (55g)
Servings Per Container About 8

Amount Per Serving

Calories 230	Calories from Fat 72
	% Daily Value*
Total Fat 8g	**12%**
Saturated Fat 1g	**5%**
Trans Fat 0g	
Cholesterol 0mg	**0%**
Sodium 160mg	**7%**
Total Carbohydrate 37g	**12%**
Dietary Fiber 4g	**16%**
Sugars 1g	
Protein 3g	
Vitamin A	10%
Vitamin C	8%
Calcium	20%
Iron	45%

* Percent Daily Values are based on a 2,000 calorie diet. Your daily value may be higher or lower depending on your calorie needs.

	Calories:	2,000	2,500
Total Fat	Less than	65g	80g
Sat Fat	Less than	20g	25g
Cholesterol	Less than	300mg	300mg
Sodium	Less than	2,400mg	2,400mg
Total Carbohydrate		300g	375g
Dietary Fiber		25g	30g

New Label

Nutrition Facts

8 servings per container
Serving size   2/3 cup (55g)

Amount per serving

Calories	**230**
	% Daily Value*
Total Fat 8g	**10%**
Saturated Fat 1g	**5%**
Trans Fat 0g	
Cholesterol 0mg	**0%**
Sodium 160mg	**7%**
Total Carbohydrate 37g	**13%**
Dietary Fiber 4g	**14%**
Total Sugars 12g	
Includes 10g Added Sugars	**20%**
Protein 3g	
Vitamin D 2mcg	10%
Calcium 260mg	20%
Iron 8mg	45%
Potassium 235mg	6%

* The % Daily Value (DV) tells you how much a nutrient in a serving of food contributes to a daily diet. 2,000 calories a day is used for general nutrition advice.

Note: The images above are meant for illustrative purposes to show how the new Nutrition Facts label might look compared to the old label. Both labels represent fictional products. When the original hypothetical label was developed in 2014 (the image on the left-hand side), added sugars was not yet proposed so the "original" label shows lg of sugar as an example. The image created for the "new" label (shown on the right-hand side) lists 12g total sugar and 10g added sugar to give an example of how added sugars would be broken out with a % Daily Value.

Source: U.S. Food and Drug Administration

are similar to the Weight Watchers portion sizes, the USDA MyPlate, and the Diabetic Exchange List, with a few minor differences.

The serving-size issue hits more than cereal. Bottles of juice, bags of chips, and other snack foods fall into this trap. If the food is in a package that would normally be entirely consumed in one sitting, the representative serving size and nutrition information most likely reflects the whole bag or bottle. This is important to know when you are trying to judge how much you are eating, and if it is an appropriate amount. The mantra of (mostly) eating your fruits rather than drinking them can help you avoid the problem of the juice bottle. And if it's a snack food, perhaps you can find something even more appealing on the Med-DASH plan, such as a piece of fruit, a small handful of nuts, or a cup of yogurt. If the food is unprocessed or minimally processed, it is much easier to avoid overeating because you don't have hidden ingredients to throw off your mental portion-size calculations.

To the Market!

We have all heard the advice about sticking to the perimeter of the grocery store. This is still great advice. The foundation of the Med-DASH plan is found there. Fruits and veggies in the produce area. Lean meats, poultry, and fish at the meat and fish counters. The dairy cases for milk, yogurt, cheese, and eggs. Beans, nuts, and seeds may be in a bulk bin in the produce area. Venture inside the aisles for canned tuna or salmon. Find your whole-wheat bread. Choose some whole-wheat pasta, beans, and rice. Think about shopping the grocery store in a new way.

Produce

The salad bar can be a great source for cut-up smaller portions of fresh fruits and veggies. Many stores also have cut-up fruits and veggies near the produce section. Since one complaint about fresh food is that it can go bad before you are ready to consume it all, this is a great option to have ready-to-eat freshness in an easily consumable amount with minimal waste.

Meat and Seafood Counter

Let's hit the seafood counter first. Salmon is always a great choice, both flavor-wise and nutritionally speaking. Farmed and wild salmon are both good choices, rich in the omega-3 fats DHA and EPA, which are so healthy. Tuna, rainbow trout, halibut, and mackerel are additional great choices. Many types of crustaceans are also delicious, healthy options. Lobster and crab have cholesterol levels similar to lean meat but are very low in fat and calories compared with meat. Shrimp has a slightly higher cholesterol content but is also very low in fat and calories. And as we discussed, there is no need to fear eating high-cholesterol meals occasionally.

You can find many lean cuts of beef and pork today, since cattle and hogs are being raised to be much leaner.[1] (Although we are all getting fatter, so that doesn't seem quite fair.) These cuts are listed in Appendices A and B (pages 233 and 235). Of course, chicken breasts without the skin are very lean choices, and some people are adding more chicken thighs to their menus because they are more flavorful and juicy.

Dairy Section

When the DASH diet was developed, one group received DASH without the added dairy. They did not get the full blood-pressure-lowering benefit. That's how important dairy is to the diet. With the Mediterranean diet, most of the dairy is in the form of fermented products, such as yogurts and cheeses. Full-fat cheeses, milk, and yogurt will add more butterfat, which is mostly saturated fat, and may be capable of promoting higher cholesterol.[2] As of this moment, it is quite controversial whether you need to have reduced-fat dairy products or not. Emerging research is encouraging for being able to include more full-fat dairy in your diet. Several studies have shown that people can consume full-fat and reduced-fat milk and not increase their cholesterol levels. The calcium in milk reduces the absorption of the butterfat. High-fiber foods can also reduce absorption of fat. Research is suggesting that high levels of refined carbohydrates initiate the metabolic processes that increase bad cholesterol rather than the butterfat being the main villain. (And we are limiting refined carbs on the Med-DASH plan.) I personally use mostly olive oil for cooking, but often finish a dish with a small portion of butter for flavor. (And always real butter for holiday cookies.) If having cheese or butter on vegetables improves their flavor for you and makes you more likely to add them to your meals, that can be a good thing. Consumption of vegetables decreased dramatically in the decades after people were discouraged from using butter, cheese, and salt on vegetables. Remember that fat improves the absorption of many of the antioxidants and vitamins that are key benefits of vegetables. So feel free to maximize the flavor of your veggies with a little bit of butter or cheese, if desired.

Inside the Aisles

Find some whole-wheat bread (whole wheat should be the number one ingredient). As a reference point, a typical slice of bread will have about 80 calories, although the Nutrition Facts label will list the calories for 2 slices, as a typical serving size. My personal preference is for light breads, which have about 45 calories per slice, so you can have two slices for your sandwich but only count it as one Med-DASH serving. Multigrain breads are not necessarily healthier than whole-wheat, so choose what you like. If you are choosing flatbreads or tortillas, again, 80 calories is the equivalent of one serving. Many larger tortillas, like those used for wraps, are about 120 calories. This will sneak in extra calories, which is probably not your goal.

Hit the canned goods aisle for some canned tuna or salmon. They make it super easy to make a healthy sandwich or top a salad for a really satisfying lunch. If you like them, herring, anchovies, and sardines are other canned fish that are rich in the good omega-3 fats. See Appendix E for more information.

When it comes to dried foods, most of the time, choose whole-wheat pasta or other types of pasta with high amounts of fiber, or skip the pasta and use veggies instead. If you like rice, I am going to surprise you and recommend white rice. Brown rice has been shown to have relatively high levels of arsenic (from the soil in which it grows), so you probably want to avoid it, especially if you eat rice frequently, and especially for babies. White basmati rice grown in California, India, or Pakistan, and sushi rice grown in the United States have been shown to have the lowest arsenic levels (as of the writing date of this book). If you've never tried basmati, you are in for a treat. I think it tastes "rice-ier" than regular long-grain American rice. When it's time to cook white rice, don't wash it first. The added vitamins are applied to the surface, so you don't want to rinse them away. The same thing is true for adding extra water than is needed for cooking. Please don't. Discarding excess cooking water discards important vitamins. Use just enough water as recommended by the cooking directions (generally two parts water to one part uncooked rice).

Beans are generally sold near the pasta and rice. Any type of dried bean is great for the Med-DASH plan. Low-sodium canned beans are another good choice and make it super easy to pull together quick, healthy meals.

Dry cereals, as you know, often have lots of added sugars. Try to choose varieties with whole grains listed first in the ingredient list, less than 5 grams of added sugar per 1-ounce serving, and 80 to 100 calories. (You might be familiar with the grain reference

Cooking Dried Beans

You can use canned beans as a time-saver, but you will get better results if you prepare your own. These methods work for any type of dry beans, except for lentils, which do not need to be precooked. Here are two methods: the fool-proof, slower method for cooking tender beans, and a quick method for those times when you are in a hurry.

Hot-Soak Method

Place the beans in a pot and add 10 cups water for every 2 cups dried beans. Bring the water to a boil and boil for 2 to 3 minutes. Remove the beans from the heat, cover, and let stand for 4 to 24 hours. Drain the beans, discard the soaking water, and rinse with fresh, cool water. Use immediately.

Quick-Soak Method

Place the beans in a large pot and add 10 cups water for every 2 cups beans. Bring the water to a boil and boil for 2 to 3 minutes. Drain the beans, discard the soaking water, and rinse with fresh, cool water.

serving size from the diabetic exchange lists, Weight Watchers, or the USDA food guidelines such as MyPlate.) Cereal serving sizes on labels can be very misleading, and don't always correspond to our 1-ounce reference servings for grains. Some cereals that are denser would have very tiny servings to equal the 1-ounce weight. For example, Grape-Nuts have a listed serving size of ½ cup with 210 calories in the Nutrition Facts panel (which is actually 2 servings), whereas Grape-Nuts Flakes have 107 calories for a ¾-cup serving. For cereals that are served cooked, a reference serving of about 1 ounce dry cereal is typically about ⅓ cup cooked, and that is usually not the serving size on the label. If those serving sizes for cooked cereal seem very small, try adding a serving of fresh fruit to your cereal to increase volume, satisfaction, and nutritional benefit.

Grocery List

Following are some ideas to help you create your grocery list to stock up your kitchen with DASH-friendly foods:

Tomatoes

For the best Mediterranean flavor, I purchase San Marzano tomatoes. This isn't a brand, but a type of tomato grown in the San Marzano region of Italy.

I will confess, I don't use tomato paste. It tastes too metallic for me. I just cook the sauce longer to get a more concentrated flavor.

Canned, Bottled, and Dry Foods

- Tomatoes: diced, sauce, paste, preferably low sodium
- Beans: kidney, white, pinto, black, chickpeas (garbanzo beans), preferably with low sodium
- Canned tuna, salmon, mackerel, herring, anchovies, sardines (according to your taste preferences)
- Low-sodium chicken broth, beef broth, and vegetable broth
- Extra virgin olive oil, canola oil, balsamic vinegar, red wine vinegar, lemon juice, lime juice
- Salad dressings—If you don't make your own, please use "real" salad dressings, not low-fat or non-fat varieties. The oil in the dressings helps provide satiety with your meal and helps with absorption of vitamins and antioxidants.

- Olives—We don't want to overdo these, but they are so Mediterranean, and rich in olive oil (of course!).
- Mustard, ketchup

Dry Foods

- Lentils and other types of dried beans—Lentils cook up quite quickly, whereas most other dried beans will need hours to soften.

Canola Oil

Canola oil is best for high-temperature cooking, such as stir-frying, since it has a higher smoke point. Make sure to use the hood (or exhaust fan) over your stove, because if any smoke is generated when cooking with oil, it is hazardous. The smoke contains acrylamide, which is a carcinogen.

If you don't want to spend that much time preparing, buy canned beans. (See my tips for cooking dried beans on page 161.)
- Rice—Reminder: Basmati rice and California sushi rice are the lowest in arsenic from the soil; brown rice will have higher arsenic levels.
- Quinoa
- Whole-wheat pasta—Other choices include gluten-free or bean-based pastas.
- Oatmeal, unsweetened—Be careful of individual serving packages, which may contain several times the Med-DASH recommended serving size. One serving is 1 ounce dry oatmeal.
- High-fiber cereals with about 5 grams or less of added sugar (as listed on the Nutrition Facts panel)—An exception to this is Raisin Bran: Count this as 1 grain plus 1 fruit serving. Be careful about some of the packaged "single-serving" bowls, which usually have 2 to 3 times the recommended portion size.

- Whole-wheat bread, including "light" or "lite" kinds—Light breads are either thinner cut or have more air in them. It's an easy way to avoid overeating starchy foods, even if they are whole grains.
- Nuts—pine nuts, almonds, walnuts, cashews, and more, preferably unsalted.

Spices and Herbs

- Onions, garlic, shallots, chives
- Fresh herbs, including basil, rosemary, thyme, sage, cilantro, parsley, mint, sorrel, dill, tarragon—Buy these close to the time when you will use them, or they will go bad in the refrigerator. Even easier, grow your own—it's inexpensive, fresher, and better tasting. Some people are genetically more likely to think cilantro has a soapy flavor (a confession: I am one of those people). You can skip it in recipes if you don't care for it. I might add basil or parsley instead.
- Dried herbs and spices including basil, oregano, parsley flakes, thyme, marjoram, paprika, rosemary, ginger, poultry seasoning, sage, onion powder, garlic powder, chili powder, cayenne pepper, peppercorns, caraway, sun-dried tomatoes, red pepper flakes, cinnamon, cumin, paprika, coriander seeds, etc., as you need them.
- Specialty Mediterranean spices and seasonings: Tabil (page 221), saffron, sumac, Roasted Harissa (page 220). Note that these may be easier to find online. Ethnic markets are also great outlets and usually have much lower prices. Saffron is super-expensive by the ounce, but you only need to purchase a little. Some cooks substitute a little turmeric to give a dish a yellow color, but the flavor won't be quite the same.

Frozen

- Individual and mixed vegetables—In addition to whatever your favorite vegetables are, my favorites to keep on hand in my freezer are bags of diced frozen onions and frozen sliced bell pepper mix. They make it so easy to pull together tasty meals at the last minute. And buy vegetables without sauces, which are usually loaded with extra salt, and fats that aren't the healthiest.
- Frozen boneless, skinless chicken breasts
- Frozen lean ground beef (and patties)—Again, these will help you pull together quick meals.
- Frozen fruit, if that is easier and more economical for you than buying fresh.

Refrigerated

- Sliced meats, low sodium
- Cheeses, according to your preferences, including some reduced fat

Fresh from the Market (Don't forget farmers' markets!)

- Salad bar for fresh, cut-up items
- Lettuces and other greens
- Carrots, radishes, celery—Having cut-up veggies in the fridge makes it easy to give your kids simple snacks and for you to enjoy a healthy snack while you are preparing dinner.
- Grape or cherry tomatoes or other-high flavor tomatoes, such as heirloom
- Coleslaw mix, broccoli slaw, grated carrots
- Peppers, sweet or hot

- Broccoli, cauliflower, red cabbage
- Cucumbers
- Beets
- Fresh fruits, according to the season

Meat Counter

- Fresh fish (see Appendix D)
- Lean meat and poultry (see Appendices A, B, and C)—Do you like to use ground turkey? Check the label to be sure the skin wasn't ground with the meat. You can tell by the fat content and the calories. If you don't care for ground turkey, use 85% or 90% lean ground beef. This will still have flavor and won't be as dry as 95% lean. It's your choice. If you have something high-fiber in the meal, like vegetables and maybe some fruit for dessert, you won't absorb as much fat from the red meat.

Dairy

- Cheeses: cheddar, Swiss, Colby Jack, mozzarella, and others according to your preferences. Whole, sliced, and grated cheeses. Note that Swiss cheese is naturally low in sodium. Go easy on feta and Parmigiano-Reggiano (or American Parmesan) cheeses because they are relatively high in sodium, although very common in Greek and Italian dishes.
- Yogurt, with little or no added sugar—Flavor your own with some jam or some diced fresh fruit.
- Milk, preferably reduced fat
- Eggs or omega-3-rich eggs—I prefer the specialty eggs because I think they taste more "eggy." Another good choice is to find locally raised chicken eggs. Just be sure to cook them to slight firmness, because even home-raised chickens can transmit Salmonella.

Prepping Your Kitchen

Having the right equipment will make your life easier, whether you like to cook or don't want to spend your time cooking. It's always fun to rethink what you have in your kitchen. Still hanging on to your bread machine, but no room for a Zoodle maker? Let's look at some interesting ideas for stocking up your kitchen.

- Toaster oven. Great for making small meals or reheating certain leftovers. I use mine almost daily.
- Microwave. Always great for reheating foods or making quick scrambled eggs.
- Digital kitchen scale. Helps make it easy to avoid "portion distortion."
- Food processor, mandoline, or V-slicer. Makes it a breeze to cut up vegetables.
- A spiralizer, perhaps? (Mine is just taking up space in my pantry.)
- Pressure cooker pots allow you to cook meals quickly and keep all the flavor. They can be especially helpful if you like to use dried beans, since they cut the cooking time dramatically.
- Slow cookers, so perfect for prepping in the morning and dinnertime eating.
- A "blender on a stick" called a hand blender or immersion blender. I don't use mine for smoothies, but rather for making sauces, salad dressings, and my morning hot chocolate.
- Instant-read digital thermometer. Tells you when your meat is cooked correctly and when your leftovers are sufficiently reheated (165°F).
- Great super-sharp knives, not serrated. Make cutting up vegetables easier. Thinner blades are easier to push through larger vegetables such as cabbage, potatoes, and squash.

- If I were going to add something to my kitchen utensils, it would be a mortar and pestle for mixing and grinding spices. I am especially coveting the Mexican one called a *molcajete*, which can also be used to make guacamole—always more delicious when it is homemade.

CHAPTER 12

Problems No More!

N_o problem if you are a busy mom, work in an office or a factory, travel on the job, or work from home. You have parties to attend, you go on a cruise, you have a strict budget, it's vacation time, you have little kids. There are always sweets around. You don't cook, you like to eat in restaurants or fast-food places, you don't like lots of foods. Not to worry. You will learn how to solve all these problems, because they are real life, and they will happen. You can't wait for everything to be perfect to choose the right time to start taking care of your health. Today is the start of the rest of your life. Here are your strategies.

Prep Ahead

Whether it's your kids running off to school or you running off to make it to work on time, preparing ahead is critical. Grab-and-go breakfast foods don't have to be Pop-Tarts, doughnuts, or bagels. Stock your refrigerator with hard-boiled eggs (peeled and stored in an airtight container), fresh fruit such as berries, and some nuts. Always have some cut-up fresh veggies around for nibbling on when you aren't ready for a meal. Many moms have complained that they actually can't take advantage of this because their kids eat all the veggies. Well, this is a great habit for your children. And you need to have more of those veggies around so you can take advantage of them, too.

Instead of buying processed lunch meats, roast a turkey breast or beef roast and slice it after it has cooled. If you are doing some grilling on the weekend, double up. Make twice what people will eat so that you can pull out some healthy grilled chicken breasts or lean hamburgers if you get home late or the kids are starving when they walk in the door. Pack breakfast, snacks, and lunch the night before. Make a sandwich with the sliced beef or turkey. Top it with a slice of cheese and some mustard. Separately, bag up some lettuce and a slice of tomato (you don't want them making your sandwich soggy). Add some yogurt, cut-up raw veggies, maybe a slice or two of cheese, and some fresh fruit. Pop these in an insulated bag, and you will be on your way quickly in the morning. Prefer salad for lunch? There are many great containers with separate compartments for the salad dressing. (And make sure it isn't a low-fat or nonfat dressing. Those will not keep you feeling full long enough.)

The Coffee Shop

Skip the pastries. Have a hot chocolate (I have mine without vanilla syrup, which makes it taste too sweet, and I don't need the extra sugar calories), or have a coffee or chai latte. This gives you a serving of dairy first thing in the morning. It's great for breaking your overnight fast and revving up your metabolism. Try to avoid added syrups and whipped cream, which pile on lots of empty calories. They may taste good, but if they are a habit, check your health. Is it where you want it to be? Is your weight where you want it to be? "If you want different results…you have to do things differently."

On the Job

If you have an office refrigerator, you are golden. Stock it with yogurt and cut-up fresh fruit and veggies. Have a stash of nuts hidden in your desk. Follow one of the example meal plans starting on page 117, and you'll have everything you need to stay full and satisfied all day. If you have a variety of healthy snacks on hand, you won't give in to the temptation of the office candy bowl or the doughnuts or cookies your coworker brought in. Your choice isn't between the candy or nothing. You actually have something delicious for a snack. You have set the stage for success.

What about those office pizza parties? Hopefully you can persuade the organizer to include some salad in the order. If not, grab your raw veggies. Then plan to have one good-sized piece of pizza, and if you are still hungry, just eat the topping on the second piece (including the cheese), but not the crust. You will still get all the flavor and be completely satisfied.

On the Road

Travel seems like it could be a situation that really gets you off track. But if you have thought about how you're going to handle things, you will be fine. In the morning, even in a fast-food place, you can get some scrambled eggs, orange juice, and either a side of milk or a latte or hot chocolate. Protein, fruit, dairy. It's already a great start. Some large chain pharmacies and highway rest stops now have grab-and-go packages of some of our key foods for snacks, like cut-up fruits and veggies, sandwiches, and bananas and apples.

It is easier than you think. When you go out for lunch, think about how you can add some veggies to your order. A side salad? Some coleslaw? Are you having a burger? Maybe you don't need the bun; even at a fast-food place you can get a knife and fork. Have some fruit instead of cookies for dessert. Dinner will probably be the time when you will be able to get exactly what you want. Have a side (or two) of veggies plus a salad, and either tell your server no bread, or move the bread to the other side of the table. Leave before dessert.

At the Restaurant

Plan what you will order before you go to the restaurant. Then you won't be tempted to get off track when you're there. Choose a salad, two vegetables, a good protein source, easy on the starches. Italian restaurant? How about chicken or fish? Chicken Parmesan or piccata? That works. No bread with your salad. Skip dessert. Chinese? Use some steamed vegetables such as broccoli or peppers as the base for your meal instead of rice. You still have all the flavor, but you are having a much lighter meal. Casual American? No bun on the burger, side salad. Fine dining? Lean, protein-rich foods such as a filet mignon (tenderloin is very lean), chicken, or grilled or baked fish. Lots of veggies, and a starting salad or maybe a seafood appetizer.

Fast Food

I'm not encouraging you to go to fast-food restaurants. However, they may occasionally be part of your life. Fortunately, there are now options that can fit into almost anyone's healthy diet. Get a side salad or a main-course salad. Have it with grilled chicken or even a burger—without the bun. Most place have many options that will work for you. And remember, think about what you will choose to eat before going into the restaurant so you won't be tempted by all the scents of the cooking food. Have a glass of milk to add to your dairy servings. If they have any cut-up fruit for dessert, go for it. Just watch out for high-added-sugar options like an extra-sweet yogurt dipping sauce.

Kids

When you are making dinner, you don't have to make a separate meal for yourself. If you are making a meal with potatoes or rice for your family, don't put them on your plate (but do add an extra vegetable serving to your meal).

The most challenging situation is casseroles. Yes, they can be easy and very tasty family meals. Try to make casseroles that don't have a high starchy or creamy sauce. Make sure to have "extra veggies" on your plate so you don't feel like you have to eat all the starch in the meal. And try to avoid high-salt sauces.

If your kids don't like fish, think about making some of your own lunches with tuna or salmon salad. Or grill some chicken for the kids and some fish for yourself, and make enough so that you have leftovers that you can use to top a salad tomorrow.

Making spaghetti? Have the sauce on top of veggies for your personal meal while the rest of your family has the pasta. I promise it is delicious. And add a side salad to get extra filled up. Make sure there is some lean source of protein such as lean ground beef or turkey in the sauce. If you add sausage, just have a little, and portion out more of the meat sauce for yourself.

It's a Party!

Parties are always fun, but they're often full of risks for knocking your diet plan off track. Make sure you don't skip eating all day; trying to save your calories for the party will make things worse. Make sure you have a high-protein breakfast, a veggie-loaded lunch, and maybe some more raw veggies and nuts an hour before you leave for the party. Now you won't be starving when you get to the party. Once you're there, look for more raw veggies and perhaps some slices of cheese. If there is fresh fruit, have some of that, too. Go easy on most of the other appetizers. Focus on one or two items that look delicious and have a few of each; then you will find that your cravings are completely under control and you won't feel like the event is controlling you. If it's a party where you have to bring something, bring a vegetable tray or an appetizer that includes veggies. Bring a fruit tray as well, so you have something sweet to end the meal. You will find that you aren't the only one who appreciates these alternatives, and they will absolutely disappear.

One of the major pitfalls at parties is drinking. The best strategy is to alternate wine with water. Have the water in your wine glass, so you will still feel like you are drinking and being social and enjoying everything about the party. And you won't feel like you are missing out on anything.

Got Allergies? No Problem!

Food allergies and food intolerances seem to be spreading to almost everyone we know. The most common food allergies are peanuts, tree nuts, dairy (from cow's milk), fish and shellfish, soy, and eggs. Fortunately, the Med-DASH program is flexible enough to accommodate almost everyone. When you prepare most of the food that you eat, you have more control over the ingredients and are less likely to encounter hidden food allergens.

Of course, people with celiac disease should not eat any foods with wheat gluten or any other grain gluten that aggravates the disease. This is easy with the Med-Plan when you are choosing mostly unprocessed or minimally processed foods, and because it is so flexible. You can always make substitutions for bread or pasta with the many choices that are now available. So many people have sensitivities to wheat gluten that are milder than celiac disease, but still respond well to gluten restriction and allow you to feel much better.

Allergies to nuts, seeds, and peanuts are common and can be life-threatening. If you have one of these allergies, clearly you want to avoid any foods that could cause an anaphylactic reaction. You can get more of the same heart-healthy fats from avocados and olives or olive oil.

If you have a true dairy allergy, you might be able to tolerate alternatives such as a2 milk (which contains different proteins than regular cow's milk), goat's milk, or cheese made with water buffalo milk, such as some mozzarella cheeses. There is a longer discussion of milk alternatives in chapter 10 on page 134. Even with lactose intolerance, you should be able to tolerate yogurt and cheese, since they are naturally very low in lactose. And of course, there are tablets to help you more easily digest lactose, and milk products like Lactaid and acidophilus milk that are low in lactose.

If you have a fish or seafood allergy, you want to avoid the offending foods. You might be able to tolerate some brands of fish oil capsules. If not, get alpha-linoleic acid from other food sources such as nuts and oils, including canola oil.

Because the Med-DASH plan is flexible and relies on mostly unprocessed foods, you will find it easy to accommodate your allergies or intolerances.

CHAPTER 13

Recipes: Make It Delicious!

You are in for a treat. There are many countries around the Mediterranean, with widely varied flavor profiles in their cuisines. You are not going to see the same old thing that you have seen in every Mediterranean cookbook. You are going on an adventure.

If you aren't quite up for an adventure, don't feel compelled; you will have familiar options, too. We are just presenting lots of choices for some fun, new ways to enjoy Mediterranean foods.

Soups

* Greek Lemon Soup with Quinoa
* Lentil Soup with Sorrel
* Tunisian Bean Soup with Poached Eggs
* Spicy Carrot-Orange Soup

Greek Lemon Soup with Quinoa

Makes 8 cups, to serve 6 to 8.

2 tablespoons olive oil
1 large onion, chopped (about 2 cups)
4 celery stalks, diced (generous 1 cup)
5 carrots, diced (1 cup)
4 cups low-sodium vegetable broth
½ cup quinoa, well rinsed
½ cup fresh lemon juice
3 eggs
¼ teaspoon freshly ground white pepper
4 cups baby kale or spinach

In a 3-quart saucepan, heat the olive oil over medium heat. Add the onion, celery, and carrots and sauté until translucent, about 10 minutes. Add the broth and the quinoa. Bring the broth to a boil. Reduce the heat to maintain a simmer, cover, and cook for 15 to 20 minutes, until the quinoa is cooked through.

In a medium bowl, beat together the lemon juice, eggs, and white pepper. While whisking, ladle 2 cups of the hot broth into the egg mixture to temper the eggs (this prevents them from scrambling from the heat of the broth). Pour the egg mixture back into the pot and stir to combine.

Stir in the greens and cook just until they've wilted, then serve.

Lentil Soup with Sorrel

Makes 10 cups, to serve 8.

1 tablespoon olive oil
1 medium onion, chopped (1½ cups)
2 medium carrots, peeled and chopped (1 cup)
1 celery stalk, chopped (½ cup)

1 red bell pepper, seeded and chopped (1 cup)
1 cup green or black lentils
3 garlic cloves, minced
½ teaspoon freshly ground black pepper
8 cups low-sodium vegetable broth
2 tablespoons chopped fresh parsley
1 bunch sorrel (or 5 ounces baby spinach plus 1 tablespoon fresh
    lemon juice and ½ teaspoon lemon zest)

In a stockpot, heat the olive oil over medium-high heat. Add the onion, carrots, celery, and bell pepper and sauté until the onion becomes translucent, about 10 minutes.

Add the lentils, garlic, and black pepper; cook for 1 minute more. Add the broth and bring to a boil. Reduce the heat to maintain a simmer and cook for 20 to 25 minutes, until the lentils are tender.

Stir in the parsley and sorrel; cook until wilted, 2 to 3 minutes. Serve.

Tunisian Bean Soup with Poached Eggs

Makes 4 servings.

2 tablespoons olive oil
1 small red onion, finely chopped
1 carrot, finely chopped
4 garlic cloves, minced
3 tablespoons harissa
3 cups vegetable broth
1 (15-ounce) can chickpeas, drained
1 (5-ounce) bag watercress or baby spinach (or red cabbage)
4 eggs

In a large saucepan, heat the olive oil over medium heat. Add the onion, carrot, garlic, and harissa. Cook until the vegetables are softened, 10 to 12 minutes.

Add the broth, chickpeas, and greens. Cook for 8 to 10 minutes, until the greens are cooked. Carefully add the eggs to the soup, one at a time. Cover; poach the eggs in the soup to your desired doneness, about 5 minutes.

Ladle the soup into bowls, top each with 1 egg, and serve.

Spicy Carrot-Orange Soup

This soup is spicy and the perfect place to showcase Turkish Aleppo pepper. If you like a milder soup, use less of the Aleppo pepper. If it is difficult to find, you can substitute 2 teaspoons cayenne pepper.

Makes 4½ cups, to serve 6 (¾ cup per serving).

2 tablespoons olive oil
1 small onion, chopped (about 1 cup)
2 garlic cloves, chopped
4 cups no-salt-added vegetable broth or chicken broth
1 pound carrots, coarsely chopped (2½ cups)
Zest and juice of 1 orange (about 1 tablespoon zest and ⅓ cup
 juice)
1 tablespoon Aleppo pepper
1 teaspoon salt
2 tablespoons Greek yogurt (optional)

In a large saucepan, heat the oil over medium heat. Add the onion and cook until starting to soften but not brown, 7 to 8 minutes.

Add the garlic and cook for 1 minute, or until fragrant.

Add the broth, carrots, orange zest, orange juice, and Aleppo pepper; bring to a boil. Reduce the heat to maintain a simmer and cook for 20 to 25 minutes, until the vegetables are tender.

Using a hand blender (or a regular blender, working in batches), blend the soup until smooth.

Ladle the soup into bowls, top with a little yogurt, if desired, and serve.

Sides and Salads

- Quinoa Tabbouleh
- Grain-Free Kale Tabbouleh
- Couscous Salad
- Greek Potato Salad
- Italian Coleslaw
- Watermelon Burrata Salad
- Greek Black-Eyed Pea Salad
- Moroccan Chickpea and Green Bean Salad with Ras el Hanout
- Roasted Fennel with Za'atar
- Spinach-Arugula Salad with Nectarines and Lemon Dressing
- Rice Pilaf with Dill
- Roasted Vegetable Salad

Quinoa Tabbouleh

Makes 4 cups, to serve 4 to 6.

½ cup quinoa or super grains
3 plum tomatoes, seeded and chopped
4 scallions (green onions), finely chopped
2 bunches parsley, finely chopped (1¼ cups)
1 cup finely chopped fresh mint
1 small Persian cucumber, peeled, seeded, and diced
3 tablespoons extra virgin olive oil
2 tablespoons fresh lemon juice
Coarsely ground black pepper (optional)

Cook the quinoa according to the package directions. Set aside to cool.

Place the tomatoes in a strainer set over a bowl and set aside to drain as much liquid as possible.

In a large bowl, combine the scallions, parsley, and mint. Drain any excess water from the quinoa and add the quinoa to the bowl.

Shake any remaining liquid from the tomatoes and add them to the quinoa mixture. Add the cucumber.

Toss the tabbouleh with the olive oil and lemon juice. Season with pepper, if desired, and serve.

Grain-Free Kale Tabbouleh

Makes 4 cups, to serve 8

2 plum tomatoes, seeded and chopped
½ cup finely chopped fresh parsley
4 scallions (green onions), finely chopped
1 head kale, finely chopped (about 2 cups)
1 cup finely chopped fresh mint
1 small Persian cucumber, peeled, seeded, and diced
3 tablespoons extra virgin olive oil
2 tablespoons fresh lemon juice
Coarsely ground black pepper (optional)

Place the tomatoes in a strainer set over a bowl and set aside to drain as much liquid as possible.

In a large bowl, stir to combine the parsley, scallions, kale, and mint.

Shake any remaining liquid from the tomatoes and add them to the kale mixture. Add the cucumber.

Add the olive oil and lemon juice and toss to combine. Season with pepper, if desired.

Couscous Salad

Makes 8 servings.

¾ cup couscous
2 tablespoons olive oil
Pinch saffron (about 8 threads)
Pinch salt
Pinch freshly ground black pepper
½ cup golden raisins
½ cup pine nuts, toasted
2 plum tomatoes, seeded and diced
½ cup chopped fresh mint
3 scallions (green onions), thinly sliced
2 tablespoons fresh lemon juice
2 tablespoons pomegranate molasses

Put the couscous in a large bowl.

In a small saucepan, combine 1 tablespoon of the olive oil, the saffron, salt, pepper, and 1 cup water. Bring the water to a boil, then pour it over the couscous. Cover with foil and let sit for 5 minutes. Fluff with a fork. Spread the couscous over a baking sheet and let cool.

Once cooled, transfer the couscous back to the bowl and add the raisins, pine nuts, tomatoes, mint, scallions, lemon juice, pomegranate molasses, and remaining 1 tablespoon olive oil. Stir to combine. Serve.

Greek Potato Salad

Makes 6 servings.

1½ pounds small red or new potatoes
½ cup olive oil

⅓ cup red wine vinegar

1 teaspoon fresh Greek oregano

4 ounces feta cheese, crumbled, if desired, or 4 ounces grated Swiss cheese (for a less salty option)

1 green bell pepper, seeded and chopped (1¼ cups)

1 small red onion, halved and thinly sliced (generous 1 cup)

½ cup Kalamata olives, pitted and halved

Put the potatoes in a large saucepan and add water to cover. Bring the water to a boil and cook until tender, 15 to 18 minutes. Drain and set aside until cool enough to handle.

Meanwhile, in a large bowl, whisk together the olive oil, vinegar, and oregano.

When the potatoes are just cool enough to handle, cut them into 1-inch pieces and add them to the bowl with the dressing. Toss to combine. Add the cheese, bell pepper, onion, and olives and toss gently. Let stand for 30 minutes before serving.

Italian Coleslaw

Makes about 6 servings.

1 cup shredded green cabbage

½ cup shredded red cabbage

½ cup shredded carrot

1 small yellow bell pepper, seeded and cut into thin strips

¼ cup sliced red onion or shallot

2 tablespoons olive oil

3 tablespoons red wine vinegar

¼ teaspoon celery seeds

In a large bowl, mix all the ingredients. Refrigerate until chilled before serving.

Watermelon Burrata Salad

Makes 4 servings.

2 cups cubes or chunks watermelon
1½ cups small burrata cheese balls, or 8-ounce large ball, cut into
  medium chunks
1 small red onion or 2 shallots, thinly sliced into half-moons
¼ cup olive oil
¼ cup balsamic vinegar
4 fresh basil leaves, sliced chiffonade-style (roll up leaves of basil,
  and slice into thin strips)
1 tablespoon lemon zest
Salt and freshly ground black pepper

In a large bowl, mix all the ingredients. Refrigerate until chilled before
serving.

Greek Black-Eyed Pea Salad

Serve this salad in lettuce cups, if desired.

Makes 4 cups, to serve 4.

2 tablespoons olive oil
Juice of 1 lemon (about 2 tablespoons)
1 garlic clove, minced
1 teaspoon ground cumin
1 (15.5-ounce) can no-salt-added black-eyed peas, drained and
  rinsed
1 red bell pepper, seeded and chopped
1 shallot, finely chopped
2 scallions (green onions), chopped
2 tablespoons chopped fresh dill
¼ cup chopped fresh parsley

½ cup pitted Kalamata olives, sliced
½ cup crumbled feta cheese (optional)

In a large bowl, whisk together the olive oil, lemon juice, garlic, and cumin.

Add the black-eyed peas, bell pepper, shallot, scallions, dill, parsley, olives, and feta (if using) and toss to combine. Serve.

Moroccan Chickpea and Green Bean Salad with Ras el Hanout

Ras el hanout (Arabic for "head of the shop") is a spice mixture used in many savory dishes, and it is generally associated with Morocco, although other North African countries use it as well. Each shop, company, or family may have their own blend. The mixture usually consists of over a dozen spices in different proportions, depending on the producer.

Makes 6 cups, to serve 6 to 8.

1 pound green beans, trimmed
2 tablespoons olive oil
2 tablespoons red wine vinegar
1 garlic clove, minced
2 teaspoons ras el hanout
1 (15.5-ounce) can no-salt-added chickpeas, drained and rinsed
1 shallot, finely chopped
3 tablespoons chopped fresh parsley

Bring a large saucepan of water to a boil. Add the green beans and cook just until crisp-tender. Drain the green beans into a colander and rinse under cool running water to stop the cooking.

In a large bowl, whisk together the olive oil, vinegar, garlic, and ras el hanout.

Add the chickpeas, green beans, shallot, and parsley and toss to combine. Serve.

Roasted Fennel with Za'atar

This could be served as a side vegetable with roast chicken, steamed or poached fish, a Spanish tortilla or a frittata, or other main dishes.

Makes 4 servings.

4 fennel bulbs, quartered
1 tablespoon olive oil
1 tablespoon za'atar seasoning
¼ teaspoon salt

Preheat the oven to 425°F.

In a large bowl, toss the fennel bulbs with the olive oil, za'atar, and salt. Spread them on a large baking sheet and roast for 25 to 30 minutes, tossing once after 15 minutes, until softened and caramelized.

Spinach-Arugula Salad with Nectarines and Lemon Dressing

Makes 6 servings.

1 (7-ounce) package baby spinach and arugula blend
3 tablespoons fresh lemon juice
5 tablespoons olive oil
⅛ teaspoon salt
Pinch (¹⁄₁₆ teaspoon) sugar
Freshly ground black pepper
½ red onion, thinly sliced
3 ripe nectarines, pitted and sliced into wedges

1 cucumber, peeled, seeded, and sliced
½ cup crumbled feta cheese

Place the spinach-arugula blend in a large bowl.

In a small bowl, whisk together the lemon juice, olive oil, salt, and sugar and season with pepper. Taste and adjust the seasonings.

Add the dressing to the greens and toss. Top with the onion, nectarines, cucumber, and feta.

Serve immediately.

Rice Pilaf with Dill

Makes 3 cups, to serve 6.

2 tablespoons olive oil
1 carrot, finely chopped (about ¾ cup)
2 leeks, halved lengthwise, washed, well drained, and sliced in
    half-moons
½ teaspoon salt
¼ teaspoon freshly ground black pepper
2 tablespoons chopped fresh dill
1 cup low-sodium vegetable broth or water
½ cup basmati rice

In a 2- or 3-quart saucepan, heat the olive oil over medium heat. Add the carrot, leeks, salt, pepper, and 1 tablespoon of the dill. Cover and cook for 6 to 8 minutes, stirring once, to soften all the vegetables but not brown them.

Add the broth or water and bring to a boil. Stir in the rice, reduce the heat to maintain a simmer, cover, and cook for 15 minutes. Remove from the heat; let stand, covered, for 10 minutes.

Fluff the rice with fork. Stir in the remaining 1 tablespoon dill and serve.

Roasted Vegetable Salad

Makes 8 servings.

2 medium sweet potatoes, halved lengthwise and cut into ½-inch-thick slices

2 medium parsnips, cut on an angle into ½-inch-thick slices

2 medium carrots, cut on an angle into ½-inch-thick slices

⅓ cup olive oil

2 medium beets, halved and cut into ½-inch-thick slices

1 tablespoon Dijon mustard

2 tablespoons red wine vinegar or sherry vinegar

1 small shallot, finely chopped

2 tablespoons chopped fresh basil

Preheat the oven to 400°F. Line two rimmed baking sheets with parchment paper.

In a large bowl, toss the sweet potatoes, parsnips, and carrots with 2 tablespoons of the olive oil. In a separate bowl, toss the beets with 1 tablespoon of the olive oil. Divide between the prepared baking sheets, keeping the beets separate from the other vegetables. Spread them into an even layer. Roast for 15 minutes. Stir, rotate the baking sheets, and roast for 15 to 20 minutes more, until the vegetables are browned. Remove from the oven; set aside to cool.

In a large bowl, whisk together the mustard, vinegar, shallot, basil, and remaining olive oil until well combined.

Add the roasted vegetables to the bowl with the dressing and toss to coat. Serve.

Appetizers

- Domatosalata (Sweet-and-Spicy Tomato Sauce)
- Garlic-Mint Yogurt Dip

- Black Olive and Lentil Pesto
- Red Lentils with Sumac
- Marinated Olives
- Baked Moroccan-Spiced Chicken Wings
- Sweet-and-Spicy Nuts
- Sweet Potato Hummus
- Roasted Chickpeas with Herbs and Spices

Domatosalata (Sweet-and-Spicy Tomato Sauce)

Serve as an appetizer topped with a swirl of yogurt, as a dip for raw veggies, or as a topping (chutney-like consistency) for baked or grilled fish or meat.

Makes 6 cups, to serve 8.

2 tablespoons olive oil
1 large onion, finely chopped
2 (28-ounce) cans no-salt added diced tomatoes, with their juices
2 tablespoons tomato paste
1½ teaspoons ground cinnamon
1 garlic clove, minced
½ teaspoon freshly ground black pepper
⅛ teaspoon cayenne pepper
½ teaspoon kosher salt, or to taste
2 tablespoons honey
2 tablespoons red wine vinegar

In a large, heavy skillet, heat the olive oil over medium heat. Add the onion and sauté until soft, about 8 minutes. Add the diced tomatoes and their juices, tomato paste, cinnamon, garlic, black pepper, cayenne, and salt. Cook, stirring occasionally, for 30 minutes, or until most of the liquid has evaporated. The tomato mixture should have thickened to a jam-like consistency.

Add the honey, reduce the heat to give a slow simmer, and cook, stirring occasionally, for 8 to 10 minutes more, until slightly syrupy. Do not let it burn.

Remove from the heat; stir in the vinegar.

Serve warm or at room temperature.

Garlic-Mint Yogurt Dip

If you're feeling decadent, make this dip with 0% fromage blanc (available at some Whole Foods groceries) instead of Greek yogurt. It's perfect for dipping vegetables or baked spicy chicken wings like the ones on page 193.

Makes 1 cup, to serve 4 to 6 as an appetizer.

1 cup plain Greek yogurt
Zest and juice of 1 lemon
1 garlic clove, minced
3 tablespoons chopped fresh mint
¼ teaspoon Aleppo pepper or cayenne pepper
¼ teaspoon salt
Freshly ground black pepper (optional)

In a small bowl, stir together all the ingredients until well combined. Season with black pepper, if desired. Refrigerate until ready to serve.

Black Olive and Lentil Pesto

Makes 2 cups, to serve 10 to 12 as appetizer.

¾ cup green lentils, rinsed
¼ teaspoon salt
½ cup pitted Kalamata olives
2 tablespoons fresh Greek oregano

2 garlic cloves, minced
2 tablespoons coarsely chopped fresh parsley
3 tablespoons fresh lemon juice
5 tablespoons olive oil

Place the lentils in a large saucepan and add cold water to cover by 1 inch. Bring the water to a boil; cover and simmer for 20 minutes, or until the lentils are soft but not disintegrating. Drain and let cool.

Shake the colander a few times to remove any excess water, then transfer the lentils to a blender or food processor. Add the salt, olives, oregano, garlic, and parsley. With the machine running, add the lemon juice, then the olive oil, and blend until smooth.

Serve with pita chips, pita bread, or as a dip for fresh vegetables.

Red Lentils with Sumac

Sumac is featured in the spice mix za'atar and is also commonly found on fattoush salad (a Middle Eastern salad with mixed greens, toasted flat bread, and other salad vegetables) and hummus. The ground red powder can be mistaken for paprika, but sumac's tangy punch is distinctive. This is great as an appetizer or side dish.

Makes 1½ cups, to serve 6 to 8 as an appetizer.

1 cup red lentils, picked through and rinsed
1 teaspoon ground sumac
½ teaspoon salt
Pita chips, warm pita bread, or raw vegetables, for serving

In a medium saucepan, combine the lentils, sumac, and 2 cups water. Bring the water to a boil. Reduce the heat to maintain a simmer and cook for 15 minutes, or until the lentils are softened and most of the water has been absorbed. Stir in the salt and cook until the lentils have absorbed all the water, about 5 minutes more.

Serve with pita chips, warm pita bread, or as a dip for raw vegetables.

Marinated Olives

Makes 2 cups, to serve 8 to 10 as an appetizer.

3 tablespoons olive oil
Zest and juice of 1 lemon
½ teaspoon Aleppo pepper or red pepper flakes
¼ teaspoon ground sumac
1 cup pitted Kalamata olives
1 cup pitted green olives, such as Castelvetrano
2 tablespoons finely chopped fresh parsley

In a medium skillet, heat the olive oil over medium heat. Add the lemon zest, Aleppo pepper, and sumac and cook for 1 to 2 minutes, occasionally stirring, until fragrant. Remove from the heat and stir in the olives, lemon juice, and parsley.

Transfer the olives to a bowl and serve immediately, or let cool, then transfer to an airtight container and store in the refrigerator for up to 1 week. The flavor will continue to develop and is best after 8 to 12 hours.

Baked Moroccan-Spiced Chicken Wings

Makes 4 servings.

Nonstick cooking spray (optional)
1½ pounds chicken wings
2 tablespoons olive oil
1 tablespoon baharat or Moroccan spice blend
½ teaspoon Aleppo pepper
½ teaspoon salt
Garlic-Mint Yogurt Dip (page 191), for serving (optional)

Preheat the oven to 400°F. Line a baking sheet with a silicone baking mat or parchment paper sprayed with cooking spray.

In a large bowl, whisk together the olive oil, baharat, Aleppo pepper, and salt. Add the wings; toss to coat well. Arrange the wings in a single layer on the prepared baking sheet.

Bake for 40 to 45 minutes, until the wings are cooked through and register 160°F on an instant-read thermometer.

Transfer to a serving platter. Serve with Garlic-Mint Yogurt Dip, if desired.

Tip: If you have an air fryer, these wings can be baked at 400°F for 30 to 35 minutes.

Sweet-and-Spicy Nuts

Makes 3 cups, to serve 10 to 12 as an appetizer.

Nonstick cooking spray
Zest and juice of 1 lemon
2 tablespoons honey (see Note)
2 teaspoons Berbere or baharat spice blend
1 teaspoon Aleppo pepper
1½ cups cashews
1½ cups dry-roasted peanuts

Preheat the oven to 375°F. Line a baking sheet with parchment paper and spray the parchment with cooking spray.

Spread the nuts in an even layer over the prepared baking sheet. Bake for 8 to 10 minutes, until fragrant. Remove from the oven and let cool slightly. Keep the oven on.

In a small bowl, stir together the lemon zest, lemon juice, honey, Berbere, and Aleppo pepper.

Transfer the nuts to a large bowl and pour over the honey-spice mixture. Toss to coat evenly. Return the nut mixture to the baking sheet and spread into an even layer. Bake for 8 to 10 minutes, until the nuts are caramelized. Remove from the oven and let cool completely before serving.

Can be stored refrigerated for up to 2 weeks.

Note: I used Turkish honey from Trader Joe's.

Sweet Potato Hummus

Makes 8 to 10 servings as an appetizer.

1 pound sweet potatoes (about 2)
1 (15-ounce) can chickpeas, drained
4 garlic cloves, minced
2 tablespoons olive oil
2 tablespoons fresh lemon juice
2 teaspoons ground cumin
1 teaspoon Aleppo pepper or red pepper flakes
Pita chips, pita bread, or fresh vegetables, for serving

Preheat the oven to 400°F.

Prick the sweet potatoes in a few places with a small, sharp knife and place them on a baking sheet. Roast until cooked through, about 1 hour, then set aside to cool. Peel the sweet potatoes and put the flesh in a blender or food processor.

Add the chickpeas, garlic, olive oil, lemon juice, cumin, and ⅓ cup water. Blend until smooth. Add the Aleppo pepper.

Serve with pita chips, pita bread, or as a dip for fresh vegetables.

Tip: Use leftover hummus as a sandwich spread.

Roasted Chickpeas with Herbs and Spices

Makes 1⅓ cups, to serve 4 as appetizer.

1 (15-ounce) can chickpeas, drained and rinsed
1 tablespoon olive oil
1 teaspoon za'atar
½ teaspoon ground sumac
1 teaspoon Aleppo pepper
1 teaspoon brown sugar
½ teaspoon kosher salt
2 tablespoons chopped fresh parsley

Preheat the oven to 350°F.

Spread the chickpeas in an even layer on an ungreased rimmed baking sheet and bake for 10 minutes, or until they are dried. Remove from the oven; keep the oven on.

Meanwhile, in a medium bowl, whisk together the olive oil, za'atar, sumac, Aleppo pepper, brown sugar, and salt until well combined.

Add the warm chickpeas to the oil-spice mixture and stir until they are completely coated. Return the chickpeas to the baking sheet and spread them into an even layer. Bake for 10 to 12 minutes more, until fragrant.

Transfer the chickpeas to a serving bowl, toss with the parsley, and serve.

Entrées

* Shakshuka, Italian Style
* Spanish-Style Pan-Roasted Cod
* Pollo alla Griglio
* Sautéed Chicken with Tomatoes over Haricots Verts
* Salmon Niçoise Salad with Dijon-Chive Dressing

* Roasted Cauliflower Steaks with Chermoula
* Black-Eyed Pea Falafel
* Tortilla Española
* Lamb Tagine (alternatively made with ground turkey or ground beef)
* Tabil-Spiced Pork Tenderloin with White Beans and Harissa
* Rice-Free Paella-Style Skillet
* Chicken and Shrimp Paella
* Chicken and Chickpea Skillet with Berbere Spice
* The Best Spaghetti Sauce
* Moroccan Cauliflower Pizza
* Herb-Marinated Grilled Lamb Loin Chops
* Besteeya (Moroccan-Style Lamb Pie) (alternatively made with ground turkey or ground beef)

Shakshuka, Italian Style

Makes 4 servings.

3 tablespoons olive oil
1 small red onion, diced
1 teaspoon red pepper flakes
3 garlic cloves, minced
1 tablespoon Italian seasoning
8 ounces sliced mushrooms
1 (28-ounce) can crushed tomatoes
6 cups baby spinach
4 eggs
Crusty bread or cooked polenta, for serving
1 tablespoon chopped fresh parsley (optional)

In a 10-inch skillet, heat the olive oil over medium heat. Add the onion and cook, stirring occasionally, for 5 to 6 minutes, being careful not to let it burn. Add the red pepper flakes, garlic, Italian seasoning, and mushrooms. Cook for 5 minutes, or until the mushrooms start to release their water.

Add tomatoes with their juices and cook, stirring, for 8 to 10 minutes. Add the spinach and stir until the leaves wilt into the sauce.

Make four wells in the tomato mixture for the eggs. Crack an egg into each well. Season with salt and black pepper. Cover the pan and cook for 8 to 10 minutes, or the whites are cooked but the yolks remain soft.

Serve immediately over crusty bread or polenta, sprinkled with the parsley, if desired.

Spanish-Style Pan-Roasted Cod

Makes 4 servings.

4 tablespoons olive oil
8 garlic cloves, minced
½ small onion, finely chopped
½ pound small red or new potatoes, quartered
1 (14.5-ounce) can low-sodium diced tomatoes, with their juices
16 pimiento-stuffed low-salt Spanish olives, sliced (about ⅓ cup)
4 tablespoons finely chopped fresh parsley
4 (4-ounce) cod fillets, about 1 inch thick
Salt and freshly ground black pepper (optional)

In a 10-inch skillet, heat 2 tablespoons of the olive oil and the garlic over medium heat. Cook, being careful not to let the garlic burn, until it becomes fragrant, 1 to 2 minutes.

Raise the temperature to medium-high heat, and add the onion, potatoes, tomatoes with their juices, olives, and 3 tablespoons of the parsley. Bring to a boil. Reduce the heat to maintain a simmer, cover, and cook for 15 to 18 minutes, until the potatoes are tender. Transfer the mixture from the skillet to a large bowl; keep warm. Wipe out the skillet and return it to the stovetop.

Heat the remaining 2 tablespoons olive oil in the skillet over medium-high heat. Season the cod with salt and pepper, if desired, and add it to the pan. Cook for 2 to 3 minutes, then carefully flip the fish and cook for 2 to 3 minutes more, until the fish flakes easily with a fork.

Divide the tomato mixture evenly among four plates and top each with a cod fillet. Sprinkle evenly with the remaining 1 tablespoon parsley and serve.

Pollo alla Griglio

Makes 4 servings.

4 boneless, skinless chicken breasts, about 1 pound
3 tablespoons olive oil
1 garlic clove, minced
1½ teaspoons poultry seasoning, or a small handful of fresh rosemary, sage, and basil, minced
1 cup low-sodium chicken broth
2 tablespoons fresh lemon juice
1 tablespoon butter
Freshly ground black pepper
Mixed greens, for serving
2 cups cherry or grape tomatoes, halved, for serving

Preheat the oven to 400°F.

In a small bowl, whisk together 2 tablespoons of the olive oil, the garlic, and the poultry seasoning. Put the chicken in a large zip-top plastic bag and pour in the marinade. Seal the bag and turn to coat the chicken. Refrigerate for 30 minutes.

Heat a grill to medium or heat a large sauté pan over medium-high heat.

Grill or cook the chicken for 4 minutes on each side, or until browned. Transfer the chicken to a plate and cover. In the same pan (or in a large sauté pan, if you grilled the chicken), bring the broth to a boil over medium heat. Add the remaining 1 tablespoon olive oil, the lemon juice, and the butter and season with pepper. Cook for 5 minutes, then return the chicken to the pan and cook, turning the chicken to coat with the sauce, for 3 to 4 minutes.

Mound some mixed greens on each of four plates. Divide the tomatoes among the plates and top each with one chicken breast. Spoon some of the sauce on top of each.

Sautéed Chicken with Tomatoes over Haricots Verts

This recipe idea was inspired by foods we had on hand, including our garden bounty. It was a great way to utilize the excess Super Sweet 100 mini cherry tomatoes from the garden. It makes a lovely meal, whether you're using ingredients pulled together from your garden or from the market.

Makes 4 servings.

2 tablespoons olive oil
8 thin-cut boneless, skinless chicken breasts
3 cups haricots verts (very thin whole green beans)
2 cups cherry or grape tomatoes, halved
1 or 2 garlic cloves, minced or pressed (½ teaspoon; optional)
1 medium onion, diced, or 1 cup frozen diced onions
1 small handful of mixed fresh parsley, oregano, and basil, minced, or 2 teaspoons Italian seasoning
½ cup low-sodium chicken broth or white wine

Preheat the oven (or a toaster oven) to 250°F.

In a large nonstick skillet, heat the olive oil over medium-high heat in a nonstick skillet. Working in batches as needed (you may only be able to do 2 to 4 breasts at a time, depending on the size of your skillet), add the chicken and cook for 1 minute, then reduce the heat to medium and cook for 2 to 3 minutes more. Turn the breast and cook for 2 minutes more, until browned on both sides but not cooked through (the chicken will finish cooking in the sauce). Remove and place on baking sheet in oven or transfer the chicken to a platter and cover to keep warm. Repeat until you have cooked all the chicken.

Immediately start cooking the green beans in a microwave or in a steamer basket over a pot of boiling water for about 5 minutes, or until crisp-tender.

In the same skillet, sauté the tomatoes, garlic (if using), and frozen diced onions (no need to thaw them first) over medium-low heat. Add the herbs and the broth and cook until the liquid has reduced and thickened slightly. Return all the chicken to the skillet and spoon the sauce over the chicken.

Divide the haricots verts among four plates. Place two chicken breasts on top of the beans on each plate, top with the sauce, and serve.

Salmon Niçoise Salad with Dijon-Chive Dressing

Makes 4 servings.

1 pound baby or fingerling potatoes
½ pound green beans
6 tablespoons olive oil
4 (4-ounce) salmon fillets
¼ teaspoon freshly ground black pepper
2 teaspoons Dijon mustard
3 tablespoons red wine vinegar
1 tablespoon, plus 1 teaspoon finely chopped fresh chives
1 head romaine lettuce, sliced cross-wise
2 hard-boiled eggs, quartered
¼ cup Niçoise or other small black olives
1 cup cherry tomatoes, quartered

Put potatoes in a large saucepan and add cold water to cover. Bring the water to a boil, then reduce the heat to maintain a simmer and cook for 12 to 15 minutes, until fork-tender. Drain and set aside until cool enough to handle, then cut into cubes. Set aside.

Meanwhile, bring a medium saucepan of water to a boil. Add the green beans and cook for 3 minutes. Drain and rinse with cold water to stop the cooking. Set aside.

In a large skillet, heat 1 tablespoon of the olive oil over medium-high heat. Season the salmon with pepper. Add the salmon to the pan and cook for 4 to 5 minutes on each side. Transfer to a platter; keep warm.

In a small bowl, whisk together the mustard, vinegar, 1 tablespoon of chives, and remaining 5 tablespoons olive oil.

Divide the lettuce evenly among four plates. Add 1 salmon fillet to each plate. Divide the potatoes, green beans, eggs, olives, and tomatoes among the plates and drizzle with the dressing. Sprinkle with the remaining 1 teaspoon chives and serve.

Roasted Cauliflower Steaks with Chermoula

This recipe makes slightly more chermoula than you'll need for four servings. Use the leftovers for topping chicken breasts or mild-flavored grilled fish, such as tilapia. It will keep in an airtight container in the refrigerator for 2 to 3 days. Bring to room temperature before using.

Makes 4 servings.

Olive oil cooking spray (optional)
½ cup olive oil, plus more for the pan if needed
1 large head cauliflower
Zest and juice of 1 small lemon
¼ cup chopped fresh parsley
¼ cup chopped fresh cilantro
5 garlic cloves, minced

1 teaspoon ground cumin
¼ teaspoon cayenne pepper
¼ teaspoon salt

Preheat the oven to 425°F. Lightly brush a baking sheet with olive oil or spray with olive oil cooking spray.

Slice the cauliflower into 1½-inch-thick slabs through the stem. Lay the slabs on the prepared baking sheet and drizzle them evenly with a scant 3 tablespoons of the olive oil. Sprinkle with pepper, if desired. Roast for 30 minutes, turning once halfway through the cooking time.

Meanwhile, in a small bowl, whisk together the lemon zest, lemon juice, parsley, cilantro, garlic, cumin, cayenne, and remaining olive oil until well combined.

Serve the cauliflower topped with the chermoula.

Black-Eyed Pea Falafel

Falafel patties can be made ahead. Serve with heated whole-wheat pitas, your favorite yogurt sauce or tahini, fresh chopped cucumbers, sliced red onions, and tomatoes.

Makes 12 patties, to serve 4.

1 (15.5-ounce) can black-eyed peas, drained
1 egg
1 tablespoon all-purpose flour
¾ cup chopped fresh parsley
¾ cup chopped fresh cilantro
5 garlic cloves, minced
1 teaspoon ground cumin
½ teaspoon red pepper flakes (optional)
⅛ teaspoon ground cinnamon
2 tablespoons olive oil

Line a baking sheet with paper towels. Spread the black-eyed peas over the prepared baking sheet and let rest for 15 minutes or longer to remove moisture.

Transfer the black-eyed peas to a food processor and pulse until coarsely ground; do not puree them.

In a large bowl, whisk together the egg and flour until well combined. Stir in the parsley, cilantro, garlic, cumin, red pepper flakes (if using), and cinnamon. Add the black-eyed peas. Mix well to evenly distribute all the ingredients. Transfer the mixture to a bowl, cover, and refrigerate for at least 30 minutes or up to overnight.

Shape the chilled mixture into twelve 2-inch patties.

In a 10-inch nonstick skillet, heat 1 tablespoon of the olive oil (see Note) over medium-high heat. In batches, add the falafel patties and cook for 3 minutes on each side, or until browned on both sides. Add the remaining 1 tablespoon olive oil, if necessary for subsequent batches.

Note: The falafel patties will absorb as much oil as you use in the pan, so do not add all the oil to start.

Tortilla Española

Spanish tortillas are more like frittatas, not a flat bread. Great for an easy light family dinner.

Makes 6 servings.

2 small potatoes (10 ounces) or mushrooms
1 red bell pepper cut in half lengthwise
⅓ cup finely chopped onion
2 tablespoons olive oil
1 garlic clove, minced
½ teaspoon red pepper flakes

6 eggs
½ teaspoon salt
1 tablespoon chopped fresh parsley

Put the potatoes in a medium saucepan, and cover with cold water by 2 inches. Bring to a boil. Reduce the heat and simmer until the potatoes are just tender. Let the potatoes cool, then peel and dice them (you should have about 1½ cups).

Preheat oven to 450°F. Put the pepper halves, cut side down, on a baking sheet lined with parchment paper. Roast for about 20 minutes, or until charred. Put the roasted pepper in a bowl and cover with plastic wrap; set aside for 15 minutes. Peel, seed, and finely chop the pepper (you should have about 1 cup).

In an 8-inch skillet, heat the olive oil over medium-high heat. Add the onion and garlic. Cook, stirring, for 1 to 2 minutes, until the onion begins to soften. Reduce the heat to medium and add the potatoes, roasted pepper, and red pepper flakes. Cook for 2 to 3 minutes, until the potatoes begin to brown.

In a small bowl, whisk the eggs and salt. Reduce the heat under the skillet to medium-low and pour in the eggs. Cover with a lid and cook for 12 to 15 minutes. Remove the skillet from heat. Turn the omelet out onto a serving platter and let cool for 10 to 15 minutes.

Sprinkle with the parsley. Slice and serve.

Lamb Tagine

Serve over cooked couscous, quinoa, or rice.

Makes 8 servings.

1 teaspoon smoked paprika
1 teaspoon ground turmeric
1 teaspoon ground cinnamon

½ teaspoon ground ginger
½ teaspoon Aleppo pepper or red pepper flakes
2 pounds boneless leg of lamb, cut into 2-inch pieces
3 tablespoons olive oil
1 large onion, chopped (about 2 cups)
4 garlic cloves, minced
1 cup low-sodium chicken broth
3 tablespoons honey, preferable Turkish (see Note)
1 pound carrots, cut into ½-inch pieces
6 ounces dried apricots

In a large bowl, combine the smoked paprika, turmeric, cinnamon, and Aleppo pepper. Add the lamb; toss to coat well.

In a large Dutch oven or tagine, heat 1 tablespoon of the olive oil. Add half the meat and cook, turning occasionally, for 5 minutes, or until evenly browned. Transfer the meat to a plate. Repeat with a second tablespoon of the olive oil and the remaining lamb.

Add the remaining 1 tablespoon olive oil to the pot. Add the onion and cook, stirring frequently, for 5 minutes. Add the broth and honey; stir. Return the lamb and any accumulated juices from the plate to the pot. Stir in the carrots and apricots. Raise the heat to high and bring to a boil. Reduce the heat to medium-low, cover, and simmer for 1 hour 15 minutes to 1 hour 30 minutes, until the meat is tender.

Serve with couscous or rice, or with crusty bread.

Note: I used Turkish honey from Trader Joe's.

Note: Alternatively, braise the lamb: Preheat the oven to 350°F. Assemble the dish as directed, but cover the pot and transfer it to the oven after browning the meat. Braise for 1 hour 30 minutes.

Tabil-Spiced Pork Tenderloin with White Beans and Harissa

If you are used to cooking pork until its internal temperature is 165°F, you will be surprised at how tender this dish is. The new guidelines from the USDA recommend cooking pork to an internal temperature of 145°F, and when you let it sit for 10 minutes after cooking, the temperature will rise further to about 155°F. By not overcooking the dish, you'll make it much more flavorful and tender.

Makes 4 servings.

Nonstick cooking spray
1 (15.5-ounce) can small white beans, undrained
½ small white onion, sliced into half-moons
1 garlic clove, minced
2 tablespoons Roasted Harissa (page 220) or store-bought harissa, plus more for serving if desired
1 (1-pound) pork tenderloin
1 tablespoon olive oil
1 tablespoon Tabil (page 221)
2 tablespoons chopped fresh parsley

Preheat the oven to 350°F. Spray a baking sheet with cooking spray.

In a medium bowl, stir together the beans, onion, garlic, and harissa. Spread the beans in an even layer over the prepared baking sheet.

Brush the pork tenderloin with the olive oil and sprinkle it on all sides with the tabil. Place it over beans.

Bake for 30 to 35 minutes, until the meat is cooked through and registers 145°F on an instant-read thermometer. Transfer the meat to a cutting board; let stand for 10 minutes before slicing.

Stir the parsley into the beans.

Serve family-style with more Roasted Harissa, if desired.

Rice-Free Paella-Style Skillet

Makes 6 servings.

3 tablespoons olive oil

1 small white onion, chopped

3 garlic cloves, minced

6 bone-in, skin-on chicken thighs or chicken breasts (2½ to 3 pounds)

12 ounces andouille or other smoked cooked sausage (such as Spanish chorizo), sliced into ½-inch-thick pieces

1 (14.5-ounce) can diced tomatoes, with their juices

1 packet saffron seasoning (0.12 gram)

1 cup thawed frozen peas

2 tablespoons chopped fresh parsley

Hot cooked yellow rice, for serving (optional) (see note below)

In a large saucepan, heat 2 tablespoons of the olive oil over medium heat. Add the onion and cook, stirring occasionally, for 5 minutes, or until softened. Add the garlic, chicken, and remaining 1 tablespoon olive oil. Cook for 6 to 8 minutes, until the chicken begins to brown, turning once.

Add the sausage, tomatoes with their juices, and saffron seasoning. Bring to a boil. Reduce the heat to medium-low, cover, and cook for 18 to 20 minutes, until a thermometer inserted into the thickest part of the chicken registers 160°F.

Uncover the pot and stir in the peas. Cover and cook for 3 to 5 minutes, until the peas are heated through.

Top with the parsley. Serve with (or without) hot cooked yellow rice.

Note: A great rice alternative would be riced cauliflower (found pre-made in the frozen food section).

Chicken and Shrimp Paella

A one-pot meal that is perfect for a weeknight but impressive enough to serve to guests.

Makes 6 servings.

3 tablespoons olive oil
1 onion, chopped (about 2 cups)
5 garlic cloves, minced
1 pound chicken breasts, cut into 1-inch pieces
1 cup Arborio rice
1 teaspoon ground cumin
1 teaspoon smoked paprika
½ teaspoon ground turmeric
1½ cups low-sodium chicken broth
1 (14.5-ounce) can diced tomatoes, with their juices
Zest and juice of 1 lemon
½ teaspoon salt
1 cup thawed frozen peas
1 medium zucchini, cut into cubes (about 2 cups)
8 ounces uncooked shrimp, thawed, peeled, and deveined
2 tablespoons chopped fresh parsley

In a large saucepan, heat 2 tablespoons of the olive oil over medium heat. Add the onion and cook, occasionally stirring, for 5 minutes, or until softened. Add the garlic, chicken, rice, and remaining 1 tablespoon olive oil. Stir until the rice is coated with the oil.

Add the cumin, smoked paprika, turmeric, broth, tomatoes with their juices, lemon zest, lemon juice, and salt. Spread the rice mixture evenly in the pan. Bring to a boil. Reduce the heat to medium-low, cover, and cook for 25 minutes—do not stir.

Remove the lid and stir in the peas and zucchini. Add the shrimp, nestling them into the rice. Cover and cook for 8 to 10 minutes. Remove from the heat and let stand for 10 minutes.

Top with the parsley and serve.

Chicken and Chickpea Skillet with Berbere Spice

A hearty skillet that showcases the flavors of the Middle East.

Makes 6 servings.

2 tablespoons olive oil
1 (3- to 4-pound) whole chicken, cut into 8 pieces
3 teaspoons Berbere or baharat spice blend
1 large onion, preferably Spanish, thinly sliced into half-moons
2 garlic cloves, minced
2 cups 1-inch cubes peeled butternut squash, or 1 (12-ounce) bag
   pre-cut squash
1 (15-ounce) can no-salt-added chickpeas, undrained
½ cup golden raisins
Hot cooked rice, for serving

In a 12-inch skillet, heat 1 tablespoon olive oil over medium-high heat. Sprinkle the chicken with 2 teaspoons of the Berbere spice. Add half the chicken to the skillet and cook until browned, 4 to 6 minutes per side. Transfer the chicken to a plate and repeat to brown the remaining chicken. Set aside.

In the same skillet, heat the remaining 1 tablespoon olive oil. Add the onion and cook, stirring, until softened, about 5 minutes. Add the remaining 1 teaspoon Berbere spice, the garlic, squash, chickpeas, and raisins and stir to combine. Return the chicken to skillet, pushing the pieces between the vegetables, and bring to a boil. Reduce the heat to maintain a simmer, cover tightly, and cook for 20 to 25 minutes, until the chicken is cooked through and an instant-read thermometer inserted into the thickest part registers 165°F, and the squash is tender.

Serve over hot cooked rice.

The Best Spaghetti Sauce

This recipe is legendary. That is, the legend is that this is Frank Sinatra's mother's recipe, and his absolute favorite. I got the recipe from my friend Peter Walsh, and he didn't leave out any key ingredients (as some people are known to do when sharing recipes). You don't have to serve this over spaghetti. I usually have it alongside green beans or broccoli. You can also use "zoodles" (zucchini noodles) for a more spaghetti-like experience. This sauce is even better the next day. I love cooking a big batch once and having several meals from my efforts.

Makes 4 servings.

1 tablespoon extra virgin olive oil
1 pound ground beef, about 90% lean
4 garlic cloves, minced or pressed
1 medium to large onion, diced
1 green bell pepper, diced
1 (15-ounce) can tomato sauce
1 (6-ounce) can tomato paste
10 to 15 ounces red wine
1 tablespoon sugar
1 tablespoon Worcestershire sauce
1 tablespoon Italian seasoning
Salt and freshly ground black pepper
1 (15-ounce) can diced tomatoes, drained

In a large skillet, heat the olive oil over medium heat. Add the ground beef and cook, breaking it up with a wooden spoon as it cooks, until nearly browned. Add the garlic, onion, and bell pepper and cook, stirring occasionally, until the onion is translucent. Drain any excess liquid from the skillet.

Add the tomato sauce and tomato paste and stir them into the beef mixture. Add the wine, sugar, Worcestershire, and Italian seasoning. Season with salt and pepper. Cook over low heat, stirring occasionally, for at least 1 hour, or as long as 4 hours, adding more water as needed to maintain the desired consistency.

Ten minutes before serving, stir in the diced tomatoes.

Moroccan Cauliflower Pizza

Makes 4 servings.

2 tablespoons olive oil
1 small onion, finely chopped
3 garlic cloves, minced
1 tablespoon Baharat spice blend
1 (14.5-ounce) can diced tomatoes in sauce
½ teaspoon salt
¾ pound ground lamb
4 tablespoons chopped fresh cilantro
1 store-bought cauliflower pizza crust
1 small Persian cucumber, peeled, seeded, and chopped
4 ounces feta cheese, crumbled (optional)

Preheat the oven according to the instructions on the cauliflower pizza crust package.

In a 10-inch skillet, heat the olive oil over medium heat. Add the onion and cook for 4 to 5 minutes, until it starts to soften. Add the garlic and Baharat spice and cook for 1 minute, or until fragrant.

Add the tomatoes with their sauce and the salt. Cook, stirring, for 10 minutes. Add the lamb and cook, stirring often and breaking up the meat with a wooden spoon as it cooks, for 8 to 10 minutes. Stir in 2 tablespoons of the cilantro.

Meanwhile, cook the cauliflower pizza crust according to the package directions. Remove the crust from the oven and top it with lamb mixture.

Sprinkle the pizza with the cucumber, remaining 2 tablespoons cilantro, and the feta, if desired. Serve immediately.

Herb-Marinated Grilled Lamb Loin Chops

Makes 4 to 6 servings.

3 tablespoons olive oil
Zest and juice of 1 lemon
2 tablespoons pomegranate molasses
1 cup finely chopped fresh mint
½ cup finely chopped fresh cilantro or parsley
2 scallions (green onions), finely chopped
6 lamb loin chops
Freshly ground black pepper
Parsley-Mint Sauce (page 220), for serving

In a small bowl, whisk together the olive oil, lemon zest, lemon juice, pomegranate molasses, mint, parsley, and scallions until well combined. Put the lamb in a large zip-top plastic bag. Add the marinade, seal the bag, and massage the marinade onto all sides of the chops. Refrigerate for at least 1 hour or up to overnight.

When ready to cook, heat a grill to medium.

Remove the chops from the marinade; discard the marinade. Season with pepper, if desired. Grill the chops for 10 to 12 minutes, turning once, for medium. Let rest for 10 minutes before serving.

Serve with Parsley-Mint Sauce.

Beesteya (Moroccan-Style Lamb Pie)

Makes 8 servings.

2 tablespoons olive oil
1 medium onion, chopped (about 1¼ cups)
3 carrots, finely chopped (about 1 cup)
1 teaspoon ground turmeric
2 garlic cloves, minced
1 pound ground lamb, turkey, or lean beef
⅓ cup golden raisins
½ cup pistachios, toasted
¼ cup chopped fresh cilantro
1 teaspoon ground cinnamon
6 eggs
1 (5-ounce) container 2% Greek yogurt
Olive oil cooking spray or other nonstick cooking spray
12 sheets frozen phyllo dough, thawed

Preheat the oven to 375°F.

In a large skillet, heat 1 tablespoon of the olive oil over medium heat. Add the onion and carrots and cook, stirring occasionally for 5 to 6 minutes, until the onion is translucent. Stir in the turmeric and garlic; cook for 1 minute. Add the remaining 1 tablespoon olive oil and the ground lamb to the skillet. Cook, breaking up the meat with a wooden spoon as it cooks, for 6 to 8 minutes, until the lamb is browned.

Stir in the raisins, pistachios, cilantro, and cinnamon until well combined; set aside.

In a medium bowl, whisk the eggs and yogurt together; set aside.

Spray a 9-inch springform pan with olive oil cooking spray or other cooking spray. On a clean work surface, stack 4 phyllo sheets, spray both sides with cooking spray, and place in the stack in the prepared pan, extending the edges of the stack up the sides of the pan. Repeat with a second stack of 4 phyllo sheets; place them crosswise over the first stack, extending the edges over the top edge of the pan.

Fill the phyllo crust with the lamb mixture, then pour in the egg mixture. Spray the remaining 4 phyllo sheets with cooking spray and cut in half. Place them over the filling to cover it completely. Fold the phyllo toward the center over the filling. Spray with additional cooking spray.

Bake for 45 to 50 minutes, until golden brown. Let stand for 15 minutes before serving.

Dressings and Sauces

Making your own salad dressings is the only way to be sure they contain healthy oils and avoid unwanted additives. And they're so easy to make. A side benefit is that it helps you use up your olive oil supply so it doesn't get old or develop off flavors.

* Maltese Sun-Dried Tomato and Mushroom Dressing
* Vinaigrette
* Citrus Vinaigrette
* Dijon Vinaigrette
* Italian Dressing
* Ranch Dressing
* Pesto
* Guacamole
* Parsley-Mint Sauce
* Roasted Harissa
* Tabil (Tunisian Five-Spice Blend)
* Sofrito
* Red Pepper Chimichurri
* Lemon-Dill Vinaigrette

Maltese Sun-Dried Tomato and Mushroom Dressing

Makes 4 (1-cup) servings.

⅓ cup olive oil (use a combination of olive oil and sun-dried tomato
     oil, if they were packed in oil)
8 ounces mushrooms, sliced
3 tablespoons red wine vinegar
freshly ground black pepper, to taste
½ cup sun-dried tomatoes, drained (if they are packed in oil,
     reserve the oil) and chopped

In a medium skillet, heat 2 tablespoons of the olive oil (or mixed olive
oil and sun-dried tomato packing oil) over high heat. Add the mushrooms and cook, stirring, until they have released their liquid.

Add vinegar and season with pepper. Remove from the heat and add
the remaining oil and the sun-dried tomatoes.

*Serving Suggestion: Toss the warm dressing with 5 cups baby spinach
(one 5-ounce bag) until the leaves are coated and slightly wilted.
Serve immediately.*

Vinaigrette

Makes 4 (1-ounce) servings.

2 tablespoons balsamic vinegar
2 large garlic cloves, minced
1 teaspoon dried rosemary, crushed
¼ teaspoon freshly ground black pepper
¼ cup olive oil

In a small bowl, whisk together the vinegar, garlic, rosemary, and pepper. While whisking, slowly stream in the olive oil and whisk until emulsified. Store in an airtight container in the refrigerator for up to 3 days.

Citrus Vinaigrette

Makes 4 (1-ounce) servings.

Zest of 1 lemon
3 tablespoons fresh lemon juice
Pinch kosher salt
Pinch freshly ground black pepper
2 tablespoons olive oil

In a small bowl, whisk together the lemon zest, lemon juice, 3 table-spoons water, the salt, and the pepper. While whisking, gradually stream in the olive oil and whisk until emulsified. Store in an airtight container in the refrigerator for up to 3 days.

Dijon Vinaigrette

Makes 4 (1-ounce) servings.

2 tablespoons red wine vinegar
2 tablespoons olive oil
1 teaspoon Dijon mustard
¼ teaspoon kosher salt
¼ teaspoon freshly ground black pepper

In a small bowl, whisk together all the ingredients and ¼ cup water. Store in an airtight container in the refrigerator for up to 3 days.

Italian Dressing

Makes 4 (1-ounce) servings.

2 tablespoons red wine vinegar
2 tablespoons olive oil

1 teaspoon dried oregano

1 teaspoon dried basil

¼ teaspoon dried thyme

¼ teaspoon onion powder

¼ teaspoon garlic powder

¼ teaspoon kosher salt

¼ teaspoon freshly ground black pepper

In a small bowl, whisk together all the ingredients and ¼ cup water. Store in an airtight container in the refrigerator for up to 3 days.

Ranch Dressing

Makes about 4 (1-ounce) servings.

⅓ cup buttermilk

¼ cup mayonnaise

1 scallion (green onion), minced

2 tablespoons cider vinegar

½ teaspoon celery seed

¼ teaspoon freshly ground black pepper

In a small bowl, whisk together all the ingredients. Store in an airtight container in the refrigerator for up to 3 days.

Pesto

Makes 1 cup.

2 cups tightly packed fresh basil leaves (remove and discard any dried or browned edges)

⅓ cup pine nuts

3 medium garlic cloves, chopped

½ cup freshly grated Parmigiano-Reggiano cheese
½ cup olive oil
¼ teaspoon freshly ground black pepper, or to taste

In a food processor, combine the basil and pine nuts and pulse for 10 seconds. Add the garlic and cheese and pulse several times to combine.

With the motor running, slowly stream in the olive oil, stopping as needed to scrape down the bowl of the food processor with a rubber spatula. Season with pepper. Store in an airtight container in the refrigerator for up to 3 days.

Guacamole

Everyone has a favorite guacamole. You can use this recipe as a starting point and then add your own embellishments: more peppers, diced tomatoes—it is up to you how interesting you want to make your "guac."

Makes about 4 (¼-cup) servings.

2 avocados, halved and pitted
1 small onion, finely diced
1 garlic clove, minced
1 small jalapeño, seeded and ribs removed, finely chopped
Juice of 1 lime
2 tablespoons minced fresh cilantro (optional)

Peel the avocados, place them in a medium serving bowl, and gently mash. Stir in the onion, garlic, jalapeño, lime juice, and cilantro (if using). Cover with plastic wrap pressed directly against the surface, and refrigerate for at least 30 minutes before serving.

Parsley-Mint Sauce

Serve with marinated grilled lamb loin chops or grilled leg of lamb.

Makes 6 (1-ounce) servings.

½ cup fresh flat-leaf parsley
1 cup fresh mint leaves
2 garlic cloves, minced
2 scallions (green onions), chopped
2 tablespoons pomegranate molasses
¼ cup olive oil
1 tablespoon fresh lemon juice

Combine all the ingredients in a blender and blend until smooth. Transfer to an airtight container and refrigerate until ready to use. Can be refrigerated for 1 day.

Roasted Harissa

Harissa is a spicy condiment used in Tunisian dishes. Making your own allows you to control the heat!

Makes ¾ cup.

1 red bell pepper
2 small fresh red chiles, or more to taste
4 garlic cloves, unpeeled
½ teaspoon ground coriander
½ teaspoon ground cumin
½ teaspoon ground caraway
1 tablespoon fresh lemon juice
½ teaspoon salt

Preheat the broiler to high.

Put the bell pepper, chiles, and garlic on a baking sheet and broil for 6 to 8 minutes. Turn the vegetables over and broil for 5 to 6 minutes more, until the pepper and chiles are softened and blackened. Remove from the broiler and set aside until cool enough to handle. Remove and discard the stems, skin, and seeds from the pepper and chiles. Remove and discard the papery skin from the garlic.

Put the flesh of the pepper and chiles with the garlic cloves in a blender or food processor. Add the coriander, cumin, caraway, lemon juice, and salt and blend until smooth.

This may be stored refrigerated for up to 3 days. Store in an airtight container, and cover the sauce with a ¼-inch layer of oil.

Tabil (Tunisian Five-Spice Blend)

Typically, tabil is a combination of five spices, including caraway, coriander, and cayenne pepper. Use it as a spice rub on meat, poultry, or vegetables.

Makes 2 tablespoons.

1 tablespoon ground coriander
1 teaspoon caraway seeds
¼ teaspoon garlic powder
¼ teaspoon cayenne pepper
¼ teaspoon ground cumin

Combine all the ingredients in a small bowl.

It may be stored in an airtight container for up to 2 weeks.

Sofrito

This sauce is a mainstay of Spanish cooking around the world. Use it as a marinade or topping for pork, beef, chicken, and fish dishes.

Makes 1¼ cups, to serve 8 to 10 (2 tablespoons per serving).

4 tablespoons olive oil
1 small onion, chopped
1 medium green bell pepper, seeded and chopped
¼ teaspoon salt
6 garlic cloves, minced
½ teaspoon red pepper flakes
¼ teaspoon freshly ground black pepper
1 cup finely chopped fresh cilantro
2 tablespoons red wine vinegar or sherry vinegar

In a 10-inch skillet, heat 2 tablespoons of the olive oil over medium-high heat. Add the onion, bell pepper, and salt. Cook, stirring occasionally, for 6 to 8 minutes, until softened.

Add the garlic, red pepper flakes, and black pepper; cook for 1 minute.

Transfer the vegetables to a blender or food processor and add the remaining 2 tablespoons olive oil, the cilantro, and the vinegar. Blend until smooth.

Red Pepper Chimichurri

Serve on grilled fish or chicken.

Makes 1¼ cups, to serve 4.

1 garlic clove, minced
3 tablespoons olive oil
1 tablespoon red wine vinegar or sherry vinegar
¼ teaspoon freshly ground black pepper
1 shallot, finely chopped
1 large red bell pepper, roasted (see page 205), peeled, seeded, and finely chopped (about 1 cup)
3 tablespoons capers, rinsed

3 tablespoons chopped fresh parsley
½ teaspoon red pepper flakes

In a small bowl, stir together all the ingredients until well combined.

Lemon-Dill Vinaigrette

Makes 6 ounces, to serve 6 to 8 (1 ounce per serving).

4 large cloves of garlic
½ cup fresh dill
½ cup parsley
1 tablespoon sherry vinegar or red wine vinegar
1 tablespoon lemon juice
½ teaspoon salt
½ cup extra virgin olive oil

Put the garlic, dill, parsley, lemon juice, vinegar, and salt into a blender. Add olive oil and process until smooth. Refrigerate covered up to a day. (I put it into a Ball jar with a tight-fitting top so I can shake it to use later but it stays emulsified.)

Desserts

* Strawberry–Pomegranate Molasses Sauce
* Ricotta Cheesecake
* Almond Rice Pudding
* Apricot and Mint No-Bake Parfait

Strawberry–Pomegranate Molasses Sauce

Makes 4½ cup/6 (¾-cup) servings.

3 tablespoons olive oil
¼ cup honey
2 pints strawberries, hulled and halved
1 to 2 tablespoons pomegranate molasses
2 tablespoons chopped fresh mint
Greek yogurt, for serving

In a medium saucepan, heat the olive oil over medium heat. Add the strawberries; cook until their juices are released. Stir in the honey and cook for 1 to 2 minutes. Stir in the molasses and mint. Serve warm over Greek yogurt.

Ricotta Cheesecake

Makes one 8-inch square cheesecake, to serve 12.

2 cups skim or fat-free ricotta cheese (one 15-ounce container)
1¼ cups sugar
1 teaspoon vanilla extract
6 eggs
Zest of 1 orange

Preheat the oven to 375°F. Grease an 8-inch square baking pan with butter or cooking spray.

In a medium bowl, stir together the ricotta and sugar. Add the eggs one at a time until well incorporated. Stir in the vanilla and orange zest.

Pour the batter into the prepared pan. Bake for 45 to 50 minutes, until set. Let cool in the pan for 20 minutes. Serve warm.

Tip: Can be made 1 day ahead. Prepare as directed, cover. Refrigerate overnight. Serve chilled.

Make it extra special by topping with fresh whipped cream and zest from an orange or lemon.

Note: I tested this recipe using 1 teaspoon of Valencia Dried Orange Peel from McCormick Spices Gourmet Collection.

Almond Rice Pudding

Trader Joe's carries a dried sliced lemon product that I chopped and used. Whole Foods now stocks preserved lemons in their olive section.

Makes 4 cups, to serve 8 (½ cup per serving).

- 1 cup Arborio rice
- ¼ teaspoon kosher salt
- 5 cups unsweetened almond milk
- 2 tablespoons chopped preserved lemon or dried lemons (see headnote)
- ½ cup sugar
- 2 teaspoons vanilla extract
- 2 tablespoons slivered almonds, toasted (optional)

In a medium saucepan, combine the rice, salt, and 2 cups water. Bring to a boil. Reduce the heat to low-medium, cover the pan with the lid ajar, and cook until the water has been almost completely absorbed, 6 to 8 minutes, stirring occasionally.

Stir in the almond milk, sugar, dried or preserved lemon, and vanilla. Bring the mixture to a simmer, stirring occasionally, and cook until the rice is tender and the mixture has thickened, 30 to 35 minutes. Let cool slightly before serving.

Serve warm, topped with toasted almonds, if desired.

Apricot and Mint No-Bake Parfait

Serves 6: ½-cup servings.

4 ounces Neufchâtel or other light cream cheese
1 (7-ounce) container 2% Greek yogurt
½ cup plus 2 tablespoons sugar
2 teaspoons vanilla extract
1 tablespoon fresh lemon juice
1 pound apricots, rinsed, pitted, and cut into bite-size pieces
2 tablespoons finely chopped fresh mint, plus whole leaves for garnish if desired

In the bowl of a stand mixer fitted with the paddle attachment, beat the Neufchâtel cheese and yogurt on low speed until well combined, about 2 minutes, scraping down the bowl as needed. Add ½ cup of the sugar, the vanilla, and the lemon juice. Mix until smooth and free of lumps, 2 to 3 minutes; set aside.

In a medium bowl, combine the apricots, mint, and remaining 2 tablespoons sugar. Stir occasionally, waiting to serve until after the apricots have released their juices and have softened.

Line up six 6- to 8-ounce glasses. Using an ice cream scoop, spoon 3 to 4 tablespoons of the cheesecake mixture evenly into the bottom of each glass. (Alternatively, transfer the cheesecake mixture to a piping bag or a small zip-top bag with one corner snipped and pipe the mixture into the glasses.) Add a layer of the same amount of apricots to each glass. Repeat so you have two layers of cheesecake mixture and two layers of the apricots, ending with the apricots.) Garnish with the mint, if desired, and serve.

CHAPTER 14

Your Best Health: The Med-DASH Impact

Your Activity

Being more physically active is rewarding for everyone, resulting in better energy levels, improved mood, and reduced joint stiffness and pain. And you don't need to do such strenuous activity that you wear out your body parts and create pain, either now or a few years down the road. Did you ever notice that your friends who took up marathon running all needed to have their knees replaced about ten years later? And then it's their hips! If you are new to this game, you don't have to go full-out immediately and potentially hurt yourself. (You'll notice we're not using the E-word here. Too much negativity associated with it.)

We are not talking about doing more planks, or crunches, or lunges (unless you really enjoy doing them). Instead, the point is to do some motion that is rhythmical and has you breathing a little harder than normal. To judge the pace, it shouldn't be so strenuous that you can't talk normally. Find something that you enjoy doing and want to keep doing for the long run. Try walking. Jogging. Running, if you like. Swimming. Dancing. Exercise class. Marching in place in front of the TV at night or first thing in the morning. Some people like a social experience while exercising and prefer to do group classes. Others just want a buddy to help keep them accountable and to partner with on walks, hikes, or bike rides. Exercising in the morning is more likely to be accomplished, with fewer events interfering with the timing, but some people are late-night exercisers who do in-home activities while reading or watching television. Do whatever works for you. If you plan and set the stage for success, you will do it.

If you plan to do the activity first thing in the morning, lay out your workout clothes the night before, or pack your gym bag. You want to remove excuses for not being active. Just like with your eating plan, you want to set the stage for success.

Strength training is crucial to maintaining a youthful body. It protects and helps build muscle and denser bones, boosts your metabolic rate, and even keeps your genes younger by protecting the ends of your telomeres. Research has shown that even super-elderly people (in their eighties and nineties) can benefit from strength training. A landmark study done at the Human Nutrition Research Center on Aging at Tufts University showed that after eight weeks of strength training, very elderly people had improved their posture and energy level and were able, in many cases, to get rid of their canes or walkers.[1]

Yoga and Pilates can improve your flexibility and balance, as well as strength. Classes can be good ways to take advantage of these activities, or you can find videos online or on demand from your cable provider, or borrow them from your public library. T'ai chi is another great way to improve your resistance to falls (even though I was told by my instructor that it does not truly improve your sense of balance, which is an inner ear issue).

I'd like to share with you my favorite ways to be more active and physically fit to illustrate that a successful plan is one where you choose the activities that you look forward to doing. (This is not a prescription, just an example of some of the variety that you can choose from.) I enjoy walking and jogging on a home treadmill. I don't have to go anywhere to do it, and I can easily take a shower afterward. Music motivates me to move, and I don't feel like I'm "exercising." I'm just increasing my energy level and having fun. I also love swimming. There is something about the water that is almost like meditation for me. I love the peacefulness and even the sound of the water. I don't go particularly fast, but it is something I love to do and will keep doing. I also do strength training. I started out by following the guidelines in the book *Strong Women Stay Young*, by Miriam Nelson, PhD (strongwomen.com/fitness). Then I heard about a program that required working out only once or twice per week for 30 minutes. It involves working a range of muscles using weights that are as heavy as you can manage for 6 to 10 reps within 2 minutes. You move the weights very slowly up and very slowly down (SuperSlow or The Power of 10). I personally saw dramatic results very quickly. It made it easier to do all my regular activities and made me feel like my body was twenty-five again (or maybe even better than it was at twenty-five). I train with a trainer, because if I have an appointment, I will keep it. I have been following this program for over fifteen years and still love it. I have no aches and pains, which is recommendation enough for me. At times I did group exercise classes that I enjoyed, especially one that involved dance routines set to music.

That is my story. Yours will be different. Just decide what you like to do. You don't have to go to an expensive gym, unless that happens to make you feel good and motivates you. Or you can find a reasonable gym that is close to your home and has a price that fits into your budget. You might find that your cable provider has a channel with exercise classes that you can follow on your own schedule and in your own home. Perhaps you can jump rope in your basement or your garage (less likely to damage anything that way). That is completely inexpensive and doesn't require extra time to go somewhere. Walk around your neighborhood or on your local school's track for a half hour. At the office, you could get up and walk to a colleague's cubicle rather than texting or e-mailing him or her. A 15-minute walk around the office in the afternoon banishes the afternoon blahs, which can have you nodding off at your desk. At night, you could march in place while you are watching television—march through a half-hour program, and you are done with exercise for the day. Do what fits into your schedule, and do something you enjoy. Love to dance? Go to a club, or dance in your room at home. Like competitive sports? Play basketball, volleyball, golf, or tennis. Live in a cold climate? Cross-country or downhill skiing, ice skating, or even curling can keep you active in the winter. Get a dog; walk the dog. Get some friends to walk with you in the park on a regular basis.

Unless you are a creature of habit, you may want to mix things up to keep it interesting. If you do cardio on a machine at the gym, you can watch TV, listen to tunes or audiobooks, or maybe read the newspaper or a book, if you are steady enough. But don't be caught in a trap with only one thing to do. You want to have a variety of ways to stay active so you have a backup plan if you get bored with your choices.

Your Habits

One good habit can lead to more good habits. Buying the right foods for Med-DASH makes it so easy to choose healthfully. Preparing extra meals when you cook makes it easy to pull out a last-minute meal to reheat. Laying out your workout clothes the night before makes it easy to fit in a workout in the morning. Tracking how many servings of each food group you eat during the day tells you what you need to have for dinner. And choosing to focus on your actions instead of the outcome helps you develop the right habits for long-term healthy living.

Tracking or journaling seems to be especially powerful. In one study, people were asked to write down everything they ate for one year. That was the only advice they were given. At the end of the year, they had changed their eating habits to a healthier plan overall and had lost weight. Just because they started tracking what they were doing. The Med-DASH tracking forms available for download at dashdiet.org/forms are very simple to use; each day, you check off the number of servings from the different foods groups. This is particularly effective with the Med-DASH plan because it is based on getting servings from all the food groups. You can quickly see if you are missing certain foods and need to either add more servings from certain food groups at dinner or plan to adjust the next day. Immediate feedback.

The Med-DASH plan is an eating pattern and a lifestyle. To protect your health for the long run, you want to develop habits that you can sustain. I maintain that counting calories is not sustainable. It makes food the enemy that keeps you constantly on guard. Planning to eat a variety of beautiful, delicious foods is exciting and motivating. Let's make friends with food and enjoy eating.

APPENDIX A

Beef

Lean Cuts of Beef
Based on 3 ounces (100 g), after cooking

	Calories	Saturated fat (g)	Total fat (g)
Eye round roast and steak	144	1.4	4
Sirloin tip side steak	143	1.6	4.1
Top round roast and steak	157	1.6	4.6
Bottom round roast and steak	139	1.7	4.9
Top sirloin steak	156	1.9	4.9
Brisket, flat half	167	1.9	5.1
Ground beef (95% lean)	139	2.4	5.1
Round tip roast and steak	148	1.9	5.3
Round steak	154	1.9	5.3
Shank cross cuts	171	1.9	5.4
Chuck shoulder pot roast	147	1.8	5.7
Sirloin tip center roast and steak	150	2.1	5.8
Chuck shoulder steak	161	1.9	6

Bottom round (Western griller) steak	155	2.2	6
Top loin (strip) steak	161	2.3	6
Shoulder petite tender and medallions	150	2.4	6.1
Flank steak	158	2.6	6.3
Shoulder center (ranch) steak	155	2.4	6.5
Tri-tip roast and steak	158	2.6	7.1
Tenderloin roast and steak	170	2.7	7.1
T-bone steak	172	3	8.2

Pork

Lean Pork
Based on 3 ounces (100 g), after cooking

	Calories	Fat (g)	Saturated fat (g)	Cholesterol (mg)
Pork tenderloin, roasted	140	4	1	65
Pork top loin roast, roasted	170	6	2	65
Pork top loin chop, broiled	170	7	2	70
Pork loin center chop, broiled	170	7	3	70
Pork sirloin roast, roasted	180	9	3	75
Ham, lean, roasted	145	5.5	1.8	53

Poultry

Calories and Fat in 3 Ounces of Cooked Lean Poultry

	Calories	Fat (g)	Saturated fat (g)	Cholesterol (mg)
Chicken breast, with skin, roasted	167	6.6	1.9	71
Chicken breast, skinless, roasted	140	3	0.9	72
Chicken thigh, with skin, roasted	210	13.2	3.7	79
Chicken thigh, skinless, roasted	178	9.2	2.6	81
Turkey breast, skinless, roasted	115	0.6	0.2	71
Turkey, whole, with skin, roasted	146	4.9	1.4	89
Ground turkey, cooked	200	11.2	2.9	87
Ground turkey breast, cooked	98	3.8	1	44

Seafood Composition

Calories and Fat in 3 Ounces of Cooked Fish and Seafood

	Calories	Fat (g)	Saturated fats (g)	Cholesterol (mg)
Blue crab	100	1	0	90
Catfish	140	9	2	50
Clams (about 12 small)	100	1.5	0	55
Cod	90	0.5	0	45
Flounder/sole	100	1.5	0.5	60
Haddock	100	1	0	80
Halibut	110	2	0	35
Lobster	80	0	0	60
Mackerel	210	13	1.5	60
Ocean perch	110	2	0	50
Orange roughy	80	1	0	20
Oysters, about 12 medium	100	3.5	1	115

Pollock	90	1	0	80
Rainbow trout	140	6	2	60
Rockfish	100	2	0	40
Salmon, Atlantic/coho	160	7	1	50
Salmon, chum/pink	130	4	1	70
Salmon, sockeye	180	9	1.5	75
Scallops, 6 large, 14 small	120	1	0	55
Shrimp	80	1	0	165
Swordfish	130	4.5	1	40
Tuna, canned in water	116	0.8	0.2	30
White fish	172	7.5	1.2	77

Omega-3 Fats in Tuna Varieties[1]

Type of Fish	Total Omega-3 Fat grams	EPA grams	DHA grams
Fresh bluefin tuna, baked, 6 ounces	2.5	0.6	1.9
Fresh albacore tuna, baked, 6 ounces	2.6	0.5	1.7
Fresh skipjack, baked, 6 ounces	2.7	0.7	2.0
Light tuna, canned in water, 6 ounces	0.46	0.08	0.38
Light tuna, canned in oil, 6 ounces	0.34	0.05	0.38
StarKist albacore tuna, canned in water, 6 ounces	1.35	Data not available	Data not available

APPENDIX E

Sources of Omega-3 Fats

Selected Food Sources of ALA, EPA, and DHA[2]			
Food	Grams per serving		
	ALA	DHA	EPA
Flaxseed oil, 1 tablespoon	7.26		
Chia seeds, 1 ounce	5.06		
English walnuts, 1 ounce	2.57		
Flaxseed, whole, 1 tablespoon	2.35		
Salmon, Atlantic, farmed, cooked, 3 ounces		1.24	0.59
Salmon, Atlantic, wild, cooked, 3 ounces		1.22	0.35
Herring, Atlantic, cooked, 3 ounces		0.94	0.77
Canola oil, 1 tablespoon	1.28		
Sardines, canned in tomato sauce, drained, 3 ounces		0.74	0.45
Mackerel, Atlantic, cooked, 3 ounces		0.59	0.43

Food	Grams per serving		
	ALA	DHA	EPA
Salmon, pink, canned in water, drained, 3 ounces	0.04	0.63	0.28
Soybean oil, 1 tablespoon	0.92		
Trout, rainbow, wild, cooked, 3 ounces		0.44	0.40
Black walnuts, 1 ounce	0.76		
Mayonnaise, 1 tablespoon	0.74		
Oysters, eastern, wild, cooked, 3 ounces	0.14	0.23	0.30
Sea bass, cooked, 3 ounces		0.47	0.18
Edamame, frozen, prepared, ½ cup	0.28		
Shrimp, cooked, 3 ounces		0.12	0.12
Refried beans, canned, vegetarian, ½ cup	0.21		
Lobster, cooked, 3 ounces	0.04	0.07	0.10
Tuna, light, canned in water, drained, 3 ounces		0.17	0.02
Tilapia, cooked, 3 ounces	0.04	0.11	
Scallops, cooked, 3 ounces		0.09	0.06
Cod, Pacific, cooked, 3 ounces		0.10	0.04
Tuna, yellowfin, cooked, 3 ounces		0.09	0.01
Kidney beans, canned, ½ cup	0.10		
Baked beans, canned, vegetarian, ½ cup	0.07		
Ground beef, 85% lean, cooked, 3 ounces	0.04		
Bread, whole-wheat, 1 slice	0.04		
Egg, cooked, 1		0.03	
Chicken, breast, roasted, 3 ounces		0.02	0.01
Milk, low-fat (1%), 1 cup	0.01		

Good Sources of Calcium, Potassium, and Magnesium

Calcium-Rich Foods
Dairy: milk, yogurt, cottage cheese, cheese
Vegetables: broccoli, kale, bok choy
Beans: soybeans, tofu
Seafood: sardines and other fish with bones

Potassium-Rich Foods
Vegetables: asparagus, artichoke, avocado, bamboo shoot, beans, beet, broccoli, Brussels sprout, carrot, cauliflower, celery, kale, mushroom, okra, potato, pumpkin, seaweed, spinach, squash (winter), sweet potato, tomato, turnip greens
Fruits: apple, apricot, avocado, banana, cantaloupe, date, dried fruit, grapefruit, honeydew, kiwifruit, orange, peach, pear, prune, strawberry, tangerine
Nuts: almonds, Brazil nuts, cashews, chestnuts, filberts, hazelnuts, peanuts, pecans, pumpkin seeds, sunflower seeds, walnuts

Potassium-Rich Foods

Cereals and breads: bran cereals, Mueslix, pumpernickel bread

Meat and poultry: pork and, at lower amounts, beef and poultry

Seafood: halibut, salmon, cod, clams, tuna, rockfish, rainbow trout, lobster, crab

Dairy: milk, yogurt

Miscellaneous: coffee, molasses, tea, tofu

Magnesium-Rich Foods

Fruits and vegetables: avocado, banana, beans, beet greens, black-eyed peas, cassava, fig, lentils, okra, potato with skin, raisins, seaweed, spinach, Swiss chard, wax beans

Whole grains: amaranth, barley, bran, brown rice, buckwheat, bulgur, granola, millet, oats, rye, triticale, whole wheat, wild rice

Dairy: milk, yogurt

Nuts: almonds, Brazil nuts, cashews, flaxseeds, hazel nuts, macadamia nuts, peanuts, pecans, pistachios, pumpkin seeds, sesame seeds, soybeans, sunflower seeds, walnuts

Seafood: salmon, tuna, lobster, halibut, cod

NOTES

Chapter 1

1. G. Maskarinec, U. Lim, S. Jacobs, et al., "Diet Quality in Midadulthood Predicts Visceral Adiposity and Liver Fatness in Older Ages: The Multiethnic Cohort Study," *Obesity* 25, no. 8 (August 2017): 1442–1450.
2. National Heart, Lung, and Blood Institute website, "NHLBI Obesity Research," last updated July 2014, accessed April 20, 2018, https://www.nhlbi.nih.gov/research/resources/obesity/.
3. Go Red for Women website, "Women Fare Worse Than Men After Heart Attack," accessed April 23, 2018, https://www.goredforwomen.org/about-heart-disease/heart_disease_research-subcategory/women-fare-worse-men-heart-attack/.
4. National Heart, Lung, and Blood Institute website, The Heart Truth Program Materials and Resources, Fact Sheets, accessed April 21, 2018, https://www.nhlbi.nih.gov/health/educational/hearttruth/materials/index.htm#factsheets.
5. A.V. Chobanian, G.L. Bakris, H.R. Black, et al., "The Seventh Report of the Joint National Committee on Prevention, Detection, Evaluation, and Treatment of High Blood Pressure," *Hypertension* 42, no. 6 (December 2003): 1206–1252.
6. P.A. James, S. Oparil, B.L. Carter, et al., "Evidence-Based Guideline for the Management of High Blood Pressure in Adults: Report from the Panel Members Appointed to the Eighth Joint National Committee (JNC 8)," *JAMA* 311, no. 5 (2014): 507–520.

7. L.J. Appel, T.J. Moore, E. Obarzanek, et al., "A Clinical Trial of the Effects of Dietary Patterns on Blood Pressure. DASH Collaborative Research Group," *New England Journal of Medicine* 336, no. 16 (1997): 1117–1124.

8. Appel et al., "A Clinical Trial of the Effects of Dietary Patterns on Blood Pressure."

9. S.M. Grundy, "Comparison of Monounsaturated Fatty Acids and Carbohydrates for Lowering Plasma Cholesterol," *New England Journal of Medicine* 314, (1986): 745–748.

10. R.P. Mensink, M.B. Katan, "Effect of Monounsaturated Fatty Acids Versus Complex Carbohydrates on High-Density Lipoproteins in Healthy Men and Women," *Lancet* 1, no. 8525 (1987): 122–125.

11. L.E. O'Connor, D. Paddon-Jones, A.J. Wright, and W.W. Campbell, "A Mediterranean-Style Eating Pattern with Lean, Unprocessed Red Meat Has Cardiometabolic Benefits for Adults Who Are Overweight or Obese in a Randomized, Crossover, Controlled Feeding Trial," *American Journal of Clinical Nutrition* 108, no. 1 (July 1, 2018): 33–40.

Chapter 2

1. L.J. Appel, F.M. Sacks, V.J. Carey, et al., "Effects of Protein, Monounsaturated Fat, and Carbohydrate Intake on Blood Pressure and Serum Lipids: Results of the Omni Heart Randomized Trial," *JAMA* 294, no. 19 (2005): 2455–2464.

2. E.J. Benjamin, S.S. Virani, C.W. Callaway, et al., "Heart Disease and Stroke Statistics—2018 Update: A Report from the American Heart Association," *Circulation* 137, no. 12 (March 2018): e67–e492.

3. M. Aguilar, T. Bhuket, S. Torres, et al., "Prevalence of the Metabolic Syndrome in the United States, 2003–2012," *JAMA* 313, no. 19 (2015): 1973–1974.

4. B.J. Webber, P.G. Seguin, D.G. Burnett, et al., "Prevalence of and Risk Factors for Autopsy-Determined Atherosclerosis Among US Service Members, 2001–2011," *JAMA* 308, no. 24 (December 26, 2012): 2577–2583.

5. W. Insull, Jr., "The Pathology of Atherosclerosis: Plaque Development and Plaque Responses to Medical Treatment," *American Journal of Medicine* 122, no. 1S (January 2009): S3–S14.

6. J.J.B. Anderson, B. Kruszka, J.A.C. Delaney, et al., "Calcium Intake from Diet and Supplements and the Risk of Coronary Artery Calcification and Its Progression Among Older Adults: 10-Year Follow-Up of the Multi-Ethnic Study of Atherosclerosis (MESA)," *Journal of the American Heart Association* 5, no. 10 (2016): e003815.

7. M. Ruscica, C. Macchi, B. Morlotti, et al., "Statin Therapy and Related Risk of New-Onset Type 2 Diabetes Mellitus," *European Journal of Internal Medicine* 25, no. 5 (June 2014): 401–6, DOI: 10.1016/j.ejim.2014.03.003.

8. The American Heart Association website, "Symptoms and Diagnosis of Metabolic Syndrome," last reviewed July 31, 2016, https://www.heart.org/en /health-topics/metabolic-syndrome/symptoms-and-diagnosis-of-metabolic -syndrome.

9. K.G. Alberti, P. Zimmet, J. Shaw, et al., International Diabetes Federation website, "Metabolic Syndrome: The IDF Consensus Worldwide Definition of Metabolic Syndrome," 2006, accessed May 4, 2018, https://www.idf.org /component/attachments/attachments.html?id=705&task=download.

10. National Heart, Lung, and Blood Institute website, The Heart Truth Program Overview fact sheet, accessed April 21, 2018, https://www.nhlbi.nih .gov/health/educational/hearttruth/downloads/pdf/campaign-overview.pdf.

11. F.M. Sacks, A.H. Lichtenstein, J.H.Y. Wu, et al., "Dietary Fats and Cardiovascular Disease: A Presidential Advisory from the American Heart Association," *Circulation* 136, no. 3 (June 15, 2017): e1–e23.

12. E.J. Benjamin, S.S. Virani, C.W. Callaway, et al., "Heart Disease and Stroke Statistics—2018 Update: A Report from the American Heart Association," *Circulation* 137, no. 12 (January 31, 2018): e67–e492.

Chapter 3

1. N. Eckel, et al., "Transition from Metabolic Healthy to Unhealthy Phenotypes and Association with Cardiovascular Disease Risk Across BMI Categories in 90,257 women (the Nurses' Health Study): 30 Year Follow-Up from a Prospective Cohort Study," *Lancet Diabetes & Endocrinology* pii: S2213-8587(18)30137-2.

2. S.S. Khan, H. Ning, J.T. Wilkins, et al., "Association of Body Mass Index with Lifetime Risk of Cardiovascular Disease and Compression of Morbidity," *JAMA Cardiology* 3, no. 4 (2018): 280–287.

3. F. Leite, Â. Leite, A. Santos, et al., "Predictors of Subclinical Inflammatory Obesity: Plasma Levels of Leptin, Very Low-Density Lipoprotein Cholesterol and CD14 Expression of CD16+ Monocytes," *Obesity Facts* 10, no. 4 (2017): 308–322.

4. C.D. Gardner, J.F. Trepanowski, L.C. del Gobbo, et al., "Effect of Low-Fat vs. Low-Carbohydrate Diet on 12-Month Weight Loss in Overweight Adults and the Association With Genotype Pattern or Insulin Secretion.

The DIETFITS Randomized Clinical Trial," *JAMA* 319, no. 7 (2018): 667–679, DOI:10.1001/jama.2018.0245.

5. G. Livesey, R. Taylor, T. Hulshof, et al., "Glycemic Response and Health—A Systematic Review and Meta-Analysis: Relations Between Dietary Glycemic Properties and Health Outcomes," *American Journal of Clinical Nutrition* 87, no. 1 (January 1, 2008): 258S–68S.

6. F.M. Sacks, V.J. Carey, C.A.M. Anderson, et al., "Effects of High vs. Low Glycemic Index of Dietary Carbohydrate on Cardiovascular Disease Risk Factors and Insulin Sensitivity: The OmniCarb Randomized Clinical Trial," *JAMA* 312, no. 23 (2014): 2531–2541, DOI:10.1001/jama.2014.16658.

Chapter 4

1. J.M. Yano, K. Yu, G.P. Donaldson, et al., "Indigenous Bacteria from the Gut Microbiota Regulate Host Serotonin Biosynthesis," *Cell* 161, no. 2 (2015): 264–276, DOI:10.1016/j.cell.2015.02.047.

2. V. Tremaroli, F. Karlsson, M. Werling, et al., "Roux-en-Y Gastric Bypass and Vertical Banded Gastroplasty Induce Long-Term Changes on the Human Gut Microbiome Contributing to Fat Mass Regulation," *Cell Metabolism* 22, no. 2 (2015): 228–238, DOI:10.1016/j.cmet.2015.07.009.

3. T. Ozdal, D.A. Sela, J. Xiao, et al., "The Reciprocal Interactions between Polyphenols and Gut Microbiota and Effects on Bioaccessibility," *Nutrients* 8, no. 2 (2016): 78, DOI:10.3390/nu8020078.

4. The Alpha-Tocopherol Beta Carotene Cancer Prevention Study Group, "The Effect of Vitamin E and Beta Carotene on the Incidence of Lung Cancer and Other Cancers in Male Smokers," *New England Journal of Medicine* 330, no. 15 (April 1994): 1029–1035.

5. A. Abdal Dayem, H.Y. Choi, G-M Yang, et al., "The Anti-Cancer Effect of Polyphenols against Breast Cancer and Cancer Stem Cells: Molecular Mechanisms," *Nutrients* 8, no. 9 (2016): 581.

6. W.C. Knowler, E. Barrett-Connor, S.E. Fowler, et al., "Reduction in the Incidence of Type 2 Diabetes with Lifestyle Intervention or Metformin," *New England Journal of Medicine* 346, no. 6 (February 7, 2002): 393–403.

7. M.C. Morris, C.C. Tangney, Y. Wang, et al., "MIND Diet Slows Cognitive Decline with Aging," *Alzheimer's & Dementia* 11, no. 9 (September 2015): 1015–22. DOI: 10.1016/j.jalz.2015.04.011. Epub June 15, 2015.

8. T.R. Silva et al., The Endocrine Society Source Reference, "Mediterranean Dietary Pattern Is Positively Associated with Bone Mineral Density and

Lean Mass in Postmenopausal Women: A Cross-Sectional Study," *ENDO* (2018); Abstract MON-301. Report from ENDO 2018 conference, not yet in publication. The Abstract was from session 301 on Monday.

Chapter 5

1. N. Eckel et al., "Transition from Metabolic Healthy to Unhealthy Phenotypes and Association with Cardiovascular Disease Risk Across BMI Categories in 90,257 women (the Nurses' Health Study): 30 Year Follow-Up from a Prospective Cohort Study," *Lancet Diabetes & Endocrinology* pii: S2213-8587(18)30137-2.
2. A.L. Komaroff, "The Microbiome and Risk for Atherosclerosis," *JAMA* 319, no. 23 (published online May 14, 2018): 2381–2382.

Chapter 6

1. A. Goyal, V. Sharma, N. Upadhyay, S. Gill, and M. Sihag, "Flax and Flaxseed Oil: An Ancient Medicine & Modern Functional Food," *Journal of Food Science and Technology* 51, no. 9 (September 2014): 1633–1653, https://www.ncbi.nlm.nih.gov/pmc/articles/PMC4152533/.
2. J.Y. Lee, K.H. Sohn, S.H. Rhee, et al., "Saturated Fatty Acids, but Not Unsaturated Fatty Acids, Induce the Expression of Cyclooxygenase-2 Mediated Through Toll-like Receptor 4," *Journal of Biological Chemistry* 276 (2001): 16683–9.
3. J.E. Flood-Obbagy and B.J. Rolls, "The Effect of Fruit in Different Forms on Energy Intake and Satiety at a Meal," *Appetite* 52, no. 2 (2009): 416–22.

Chapter 7

1. R.H. Eckel, J.M. Jakicic, J.D. Ard, et al., "2013 AHA/ACC Guideline on Lifestyle Management to Reduce Cardiovascular Risk," *Circulation* 129, no. 25 Suppl. 2 (June 24, 2014): S76–99.

2. I. Sudano, A.J. Flammer, S. Roas, et al., "Cocoa, Blood Pressure, and Vascular Function," *Current Hypertension Reports* 14, no. 4 (2012): 279–284.

Chapter 9

1. N. Owen, G.N. Healy, C.E. Matthews, et al., "Too Much Sitting: The Population-Health Science of Sedentary Behavior," *Exercise and Sport Sciences Reviews* 38, no. 3 (2010): 105–113.

Chapter 11

1. A.M. Bernstein, Q. Sun, F.B. Hu, et al., "Major Dietary Protein Sources and Risk of Coronary Heart Disease in Women," *Circulation* 122, no. 9 (2010): 876–883.
2. F.B. Hu, M.J. Stampfer, J.E. Manson, et al., "Dietary Saturated Fats and Their Food Sources in Relation to the Risk of Coronary Heart Disease in Women," *American Journal of Clinical Nutrition* 70, no. 6 (1999): 1001–1008.

Chapter 14

1. M.A. Fiatarone, E.F. O'Neill, N.D. Ryan, et al., "Exercise Training and Nutritional Supplementation for Physical Frailty in Very Elderly People," *New England Journal of Medicine* 330, no. 25 (June 1994): 1769–75, https://www.ncbi.nlm.nih.gov/pubmed/8190152.

Appendices

1. The World's Healthiest Foods website, "Is Canned Tuna a Good Source of Omega-3 Fats?" accessed May 30, 2018, http://whfoods.org/genpage.php?tname=george&dbid=97.
2. National Institutes of Health website, Office of Dietary Supplements, "Omega-3 Fatty Acids, Fact Sheet for Health Professionals," updated June 6, 2018, accessed May 30, 2018, https://ods.od.nih.gov/factsheets/Omega3FattyAcids-HealthProfessional/.

ACKNOWLEDGMENTS

I am very appreciative of the great team at Grand Central Life & Style for bringing this project to life. My editor, Leah Miller, has really pushed to make this book a true homage to both the DASH diet and the Mediterranean diet, emphasizing the delicious foods that make it easy to reap all the health benefits. She was never reluctant to keep pushing the envelope to make the book true to our vision.

My recipe developer and true star, Shannon Kinsella, brought all her expertise and in-the-field (or should that be by-the-sea?) experience with Mediterranean foods to make this project so much fun and so delicious. I am grateful to her for helping me move this project beyond my Midwestern (and spice-free) sensibilities. I also thank her for arranging a fabulous photo shoot for our recipes with Chris Cassidy and his team.

And, of course, I am so thankful for my agent, Laurie Bernstein, who believed in this book from the beginning and wouldn't give up until we found the "sweet spot" for bringing it to fruition.

INDEX

alcohol, 55, 133
"all foods can fit," 72–73
allergies, food, 174–175
almond milk, 134
Alzheimer's disease, 59
android obesity, 32
antioxidants
    absorption of, 78
    for brain health, 59
    and cancer risk, 55–56
    and fats in diet, 78, 81, 159, 162
    foods providing, 54–55, 87, 94–95,
        97–99, 132–135
    for heart health, 34–35, 53
    and inflammation, 45–46
    in juices and smoothies, 67
    in Med-DASH plan, 90
    in wine and grape juice, 29
artificial sweeteners, 86
atherosclerotic heart disease, 27–30
avocados, 6, 34, 81

bacteria, in gut, 46–51, 95
barley, 34, 87, 88, 98
beans, 92, 160, 163

cooking, 161
    in DASH diet, 11, 12, 14, 16
    fiber in, 34, 87–88
    and hunger, 40
    in Med-DASH plan, 17, 90, 92
    in Mediterranean diet, 4, 12, 17
beef, 85, 92, 93, 158, 233–234
belly fat
    carbs stored as, 7, 41, 42
    negative health effects of, 5, 10, 40,
        41, 56, 69, 70
    and obesity, 32, 52–53
beta-carotene, 46, 54, 78, 95
beverages, 50, 132–135
blood glucose/blood sugar,
        24–25, 86
    and belly fat, 40, 41
    and cancer risk, 56
    and high glycemic foods, 42
    liver and pancreas health, 56–59
    and metabolic syndrome, 30–31
blood pressure/hypertension
    and belly fat, 5, 40, 69
    and chocolate consumption, 99
    and coffee intake, 132

blood pressure/hypertension (*cont.*)
  and dairy products in diet, 96, 133, 158
  with DASH diet, 11–15, 19, 79, 85, 93, 96, 133, 158
  and fiber in diet, 87
  and gut microbiota, 47
  and heart disease, 22–23, 25–26
  and inflammation, 48
  with Med-DASH diet, 6, 26, 61
  and metabolic syndrome, 31–32
  and saturated fats, 82
  and sodium in diet, 154
BMI (body-mass index), 38–39
body fat, 41, 70. *See also* belly fat
body-mass index (BMI), 38–39
bone health, 60–62
bottled foods, 162–163
brain health, 59–60, 80
breads, 97, 98, 159, 164
butter, 159
buying foods, 153–166
  dairy products, 158–159
  grocery list, 162–166
  inside aisles, 159–162
  meat and seafood, 158
  produce, 157
  reading labels, 154–157

C-reactive protein (CRP), 52, 80
caffeine, 124, 132
calcium-rich foods, 6, 26, 28, 60–62, 96, 134, 243
calories, 71–72
cancer
  and belly fat, 40, 41, 69, 70
  and coffee consumption, 132
  and DASH diet, 6, 13
  and inflammation, 7, 45, 52, 80

  and olive oil consumption, 79
  and oxidation, 54, 81
  and polyphenols, 50
  reducing risk for, 55–56
  and saturated fats, 96
canned foods, 160, 162
canola oil, 91, 163
carbs, 85–88
  calories in, 98
  in DASH diet, 14, 15
  empty, 40–41, 69, 70, 73, 102
  and glycemic load, 43
  during jump-start phase, 110–111
  in mixed meals, 103, 104
  and physical activity, 43
  refined/processed, 19, 29, 34, 36, 159
  stored as belly fat, 7, 41, 42
cardiovascular disease, 22–30
carotenoids, 78
cereals, 98, 160–163
cheeses, 166
chicken, 85, 93, 158
children
  complementary proteins for, 84
  options for, 173
chocolate, 99
cholesterol (blood)
  and belly fat, 40
  on DASH diet, 13, 15, 19
  and fiber in diet, 87, 88, 98
  from foods, 97
  and heart disease, 22–24, 27–32, 34, 35
  and inflammation, 53
  and milk, 97, 158, 159
  production of, 97
  and saturated fats, 79, 82, 97
  and TMAO, 93
  and triglycerides, 58

cholesterol (dietary), 97, 132, 134, 158
chronic diseases, 6–7, 9, 45–53
coconut milk, 134
coconut oil, 82
coffee, 50, 132
coffee shop options, 170–171
cravings, curbing, 36
CRP (C-reactive protein), 52, 80

dairy products, 84, 96–97, 133–134
  allergies to, 174, 175
  buying, 166
  in DASH diet, 4, 11, 12, 14, 16
  in Med-DASH plan, 90, 96–97
  in Mediterranean diet, 4, 12, 16
  protein in, 85
  to satisfy hunger, 102
  shopping for, 158–159
DASH diet, 3, 6, 8, 9, 11–16
  and blood pressure, 11–15, 19, 79,
    85, 93, 96, 133, 158
  and cancer, 6, 13
  and cholesterol, 13, 15, 19
  and diabetes, 12, 13, 35
  foods in, 4, 11, 12, 14, 16
  nutrients in, 4, 11, 12, 14–16, 19, 85
  and triglycerides, 15, 19
dementia, 59–60
depression, 49
diabetes/type 1 and type 2 diabetes, 22
  and belly fat, 5, 40, 41, 56, 69, 70
  and cholesterol level, 27
  and coffee consumption, 132
  and DASH diet, 12, 13, 35
  and fiber intake, 87
  genetic risk for, 70
  and gut microbiota, 48, 49
  and inflammation, 7, 45, 80, 82
  and Med-DASH diet plan, 58, 59
  and Mediterranean diet, 12, 35
  and metabolic syndrome, 30–32
  and nuts in diet, 92
  reversing, 58
  and saturated fats, 134
  and starch intake, 69
  and statins, 29, 56
  and triglyceride levels, 57
dry foods, 160, 162–164

"eat less, move more" (ELMM), 73–74
eating plan for Med-DASH, 89–99,
    127–151. See also jump-start plan
  beverages, 132–135
  daily meals, 131
  meal plan examples, 135–151
  servings of foods, 128–130
eggs, 84, 85, 97, 166, 174
ELMM ("eat less, move more"), 73–74
energy bars, 67–68
entertaining, food options for, 150–151
essential fatty acids, 83
exercise. See physical activity
expectations, setting, 76

family meals, 110
fast food options, 124–125, 172–173
fats (nutrients), 33–34, 78–84. See also
    specific types of fats, e.g.: omega-3
    fatty acids
  and antioxidants, 78, 81, 159, 162
  in DASH diet, 4, 11, 12, 16
  and hunger, 40
  in Med-DASH plan, 34, 78–84
  in Mediterranean diet, 4, 12, 16
  in mixed meals, 42–43, 103, 104
  oxidation of, 54
  to satisfy hunger, 35, 73
fecal transplants, 47, 48

fermented dairy foods, 96
fiber
   and antioxidants, 53
   and blood pressure, 26
   and carb absorption, 36
   and fats/cholesterol absorption, 33
   in fruits and vegetables, 42, 94, 95,
      134–135
   and gut microbiota, 47–50
   in Med-DASH plan, 34, 43, 90
   in mixed meals, 42–43
   and refined grains, 66–67
   sources of, 87–88
   and sugar absorption, 58
   types of, 87
   in whole grains, 98
fish, 79–80, 94
   allergies to, 174, 175
   for brain health, 59–60, 80
   buying, 158
   canned, 160
   in DASH diet, 4, 11, 14
   in Med-DASH plan, 17, 94
   in Mediterranean diet, 4, 17
   omega-3 fatty acids from, 53, 79
   protein in, 85
   for triglyceride control, 58
   vitamin D from, 61
fish oils, 53, 79, 80, 82–83
flavonoids, 50, 51
flavored water, 124, 132
flax oil, 81
flaxseed, 81
food additives, 55
food allergies/intolerances, 174–175
frozen foods, 165
fructose, 86
fruit juices, 67, 95, 134
fruits, 37, 94–95

anti-inflammatory properties of, 51
antioxidants in, 45, 50, 54, 55, 78
and blood sugar, 42
color range of, 101
in DASH diet, 4, 11, 14
fiber in, 34, 87–88
fructose in, 86
and hunger, 37, 40, 74
in Med-DASH plan, 17, 90, 94–95
in Mediterranean diet, 4, 16–18
phytochemicals in, 78
polyphenols in, 50
to satisfy sweet tooth, 103

genetic risk, 69–70
glucose, 57, 86
gluten, 174–175
glycemic index, 40, 42–43
glycemic load, 43
grains
   and celiac disease, 174–175
   daily servings of, 109
   in DASH diet, 4, 11, 14
   in Med-DASH plan, 90, 97
   in Mediterranean diet, 4, 17
   polyphenols from, 50, 51
   rancid, 92
   refined, 8, 58, 66–67, 69, 70
   serving sizes for, 154–156
   as starches, 98
grapefruit, 52
grocery list, 162–166
gut microbiota, 46–51, 95

habits, 230–231
   changing, 63–64, 68
   for heart health, 19
health benefits of Med-DASH, 6–7, 9,
      13, 18, 45–62

health myths, 64–66
healthy foods, amounts of, 73
heart disease, 19–35
    atherosclerotic, 27–30
    cardiovascular disease, 22–30
    French paradox, 10
    and inflammation, 51–53
    and Med-DASH plan, 5, 33–35
    metabolic syndrome, 30–35
    risk factors for, 22
    and Seventh Day Adventist diet,
        10–11
    and vegetarian diet, 14
    women and, 9, 32–33
heart health, 6, 9, 16, 53, 79–81
herbs and spices, 4, 17, 50, 98–99, 164
high blood pressure. *See* blood
    pressure/hypertension
high glycemic index foods, 40, 42
Hippocrates, 26
hot chocolate, 99
hunger, 40, 42, 74–75
hypertension. *See* blood pressure/
    hypertension

immune cells, 49, 53
immune function, 50, 82
inflammation, 7, 45–53
    and cancer risk, 56
    and fats, 82, 83
    and fiber intake, 87
    and gut microbiota, 46–51
    and heart disease, 51–53
    and omega-3s, 80
    and oxidation, 54
infused water, 132
insulin, 41, 42, 56, 58, 59, 86
insulin resistance (IR), 30, 57
intestinal tract, 46–51, 95

intolerances, food, 174–175

juicing, 67
jump-start plan, 109–125
    daily meals, 114–115
    foods to choose, 111–112
    meal plan examples, 117–125
    servings of foods, 112–114, 116

Keys, Ancel, 16–17
kitchen equipment, 167–168
Kumanyika, Shiriki, 12

labels, reading, 154–157
lamb, 85
lentils, 163
lifelong eating pattern, 75
liver health, 56–59

magnesium-rich foods, 14, 96, 244
meal plans for Med-DASH, 107
    full eating plan, 127–151
    jump-start plan, 109–125
meals, number of, 102
meats, 92–93, 158
    buying, 166
    in DASH diet, 4, 11, 12, 14, 16
    in Med-DASH plan, 90, 92–93
    in Mediterranean diet, 4, 12, 16
medications, 52, 58–59
Mediterranean DASH diet (Med-
    DASH), 5–7, 9, 11–13, 17–18. *See
    also specific topics and foods*
    buying foods for, 153–166
    carbs in, 85–88
    eating plan for, 89–99, 127–151
    fats in, 35, 78–84
    health benefits of, 6–7, 9, 13, 18,
        45–62

Mediterranean DASH diet (*cont.*)
    and heart health, 19–35
    jump-start guidelines, 109–125
    kitchen equipment, 167–168
    meal plans for, 107 (*See also* recipes)
    protein in, 84–85
    rules/guidelines for, 101–103
    and weight management, 37–44
Mediterranean diet, 3, 4, 8–13, 16–17, 62
metabolic syndrome, 22, 30–35, 40
metabolical obesity, 38–40
milk, 133–134, 154, 166
milk alternatives, 134
minerals
    in eggs, 97
    in fiber-rich foods, 87
    in fruits and vegetables, 94
    in Med-DASH plan, 26, 90
    in nuts and seeds, 103
monounsaturated fats (MUFA), 15, 79,
    81–84
motivation, 75–76
muscle, 41, 60, 84

Nelson, Miriam, 229
nutrient absorption, 78
nutrition. *See also specific nutrients*
    macronutrients, 77
    myths about, 66–74
    new eating habits, 74–75
Nutrition Facts panel, 155–156
nuts, 92, 103, 164
    allergies to, 174, 175
    antioxidants in, 54
    in DASH diet, 4, 11, 12, 14, 16
    and heart health, 6
    and hunger, 40
    in Med-DASH plan, 17, 34, 90, 92
    in Mediterranean diet, 4, 12, 17, 81

    omega-3 fatty acids in, 79, 80
    and sugar absorption, 86

oats, 34, 87, 88, 98, 163
obesity, 7
    android (belly fat), 32, 52–53
    consequences of, 70
    in Europe, 16
    and fat intake, 78
    fecal transplants for, 47, 48
    and inflammation, 28
    metabolic, 38–40
oils, 91–92. *See also specific oils*
    antioxidants in, 54
    in Med-DASH plan, 91
    in Mediterranean diet, 81
    omega-3 fatty acids in, 79, 80
olive oil, 79, 91
    in DASH diet, 12, 16
    and heart health, 6
    in Med-DASH plan, 17, 34, 90
    in Mediterranean diet, 4, 12, 16, 18, 81
omega-3 fatty acids, 82–83, 240–242
    benefits of, 79–80
    for brain health, 59–60, 80
    for heart health, 53, 79–81
    sources of, 79
    for triglyceride control, 58
omega-6 fats, 55, 79, 83
organic foods, 90
osteopenia, 60, 61
osteoporosis, 60–61
ounces, 154
oxidation, 53–55, 81, 82
oxidative stress, 45

palm oil, 33, 34, 82
pancreas health, 56–59
party food options, 150–151, 173–174

pasta, 97, 98, 160, 163
PCOS (polycystic ovary syndrome), 32
peanut allergy, 174, 175
pesticides, 55, 90
physical activity, 41, 43–44, 60, 62,
    227–230
phytochemicals, 45–46, 78
polycystic ovary syndrome (PCOS), 32
polyphenols, 49–51, 55–56, 99
polyunsaturated fats (PUFA), 79,
    82–83
pork, 85, 92, 93, 158, 235
potassium-rich foods, 26
    beef and pork, 93
    and blood pressure, 14
    coffee, 132
    dairy products, 96
    milk alternatives, 134, 243–244
    nuts, 92
    potatoes, 95
poultry, 92–93, 158, 237
    in DASH diet, 4, 11, 14
    and hunger, 40
    in Med-DASH plan, 90, 92–93
    in Mediterranean diet, 4
prebiotics, 49, 50
prediabetes, 7, 25, 30, 31, 58
preparation for meals, 169–170
probiotics, 49, 50
produce, shopping for, 157, 165–166
protein(s), 84–85. *See also specific
    protein sources*
    after exercise, 43
    and blood pressure, 26
    for bone health, 62
    calories from, 72, 78
    in DASH diet, 15, 19, 85
    in HDL, 24
    and hunger, 74

low-protein diets, 7
    to maintain muscle, 60
    in Med-DASH plan, 33, 36, 40, 90
    in mixed meals, 42–43, 103, 104
    needed amount of, 68–69
    to satisfy hunger, 35, 73, 74, 102,
        103, 110
    sources of, 85, 92, 94, 96–98, 134
    and weight loss, 70
protein bars, 67–68
provitamins, 54
PUFA (polyunsaturated fats), 79,
    82–83

quinoa, 98, 163

RA. *See* rheumatoid arthritis
rancid foods, 92
recipes
    Almond Rice Pudding, 225
    Apricot and Mint No-Bake Parfait,
        226
    Baked Moroccan-Spiced Chicken
        Wings, 193
    Beesteya (Moroccan-Style Lamb
        Pie), 214
    The Best Spaghetti Sauce, 211
    Black-Eyed Pea Falafel, 203
    Black Olive and Lentil Pesto, 191
    Cheddar and Turkey Sandwich, 147
    Chicken and Chickpea Skillet with
        Berbere Spice, 210
    Chicken and Shrimp Paella, 209
    Citrus Vinaigrette, 217
    Couscous Salad, 183
    Dijon Vinaigrette, 217
    Domatosalata (Sweet-and-Spicy
        Tomato Sauce), 190
    French Toast with Strawberries, 148

recipes (*cont.*)
Garlic-Mint Yogurt Dip, 191
Grain-Free Kale Tabbouleh, 182
Greek Black-Eyed Pea Salad, 185
Greek Lemon Soup with Quinoa, 178
Greek Potato Salad, 183
Guacamole, 219
Ham and Swiss Cheese Sandwich, 138
Herb-Marinated Grilled Lamb Loin Chops, 213
Italian Coleslaw, 184
Italian Dressing, 217
Lamb Tagine, 205
Lemon-Dill Vinaigrette, 223
Lentil Soup with Sorrel, 178
Maltese Sun-Dried Tomato and Mushroom Dressing, 216
Marinated Olives, 193
Moroccan Cauliflower Pizza, 212
Moroccan Chickpea and Green Bean Salad with Ras el Hanout, 186
Parsley-Mint Sauce, 220
Pesto, 218
Pollo alla Griglio, 199
Quick Mini Omelet, 121
Quinoa Tabbouleh, 181
Ranch Dressing, 218
Red Lentils with Sumac, 192
Red Pepper Chimichurri, 222
Rice-Free Paella-Style Skillet, 208
Rice Pilaf with Dill, 188
Ricotta Cheesecake, 224
Roast Chicken Breast, 137
Roasted Carrots, Onions, and Brussels Sprouts, 137
Roasted Cauliflower Steaks with Chermoula, 202
Roasted Chickpeas with Herbs and Spices, 196
Roasted Fennel with Za'atar, 187
Roasted Harissa, 220
Roasted Vegetable Salad, 189
Roll-ups, 115, 118, 121, 123
Salmon Niçoise Salad with Dijon-Chive Dressing, 201
Sautéed Carrots and Onions, 119
Sautéed Chicken with Tomatoes over Haricots Verts, 200
Shakshuka, Italian Style, 197
Sofrito, 221
Spanish-Style Pan-Roasted Cod, 198
Spicy Carrot-Orange Soup, 180
Spinach-Arugula Salad with Nectarines and Lemon Dressing, 187
Strawberry-Pomegranate Molasses Sauce, 224
Sweet-and-Spicy Nuts, 194
Sweet Potato Hummus, 195
Tabil-Spiced Pork Tenderloin with White Beans and Harissa, 207
Tabil (Tunisian Five-Spice Blend), 221
Tartine with Almond Butter and Banana, 146
Tartine with Cream Cheese and Strawberries, 142
Tortilla Española, 204
Tunisian Bean Soup with Poached Eggs, 179
Vinaigrette, 216
Watermelon Burrata Salad, 185
refrigerated foods, shopping for, 165
restaurant options, 124–125, 172
rheumatoid arthritis (RA), 46, 80, 82
rice, 97, 98, 160, 163
rice milk, 134

satiety, 78
saturated fats (SFA), 15, 33, 79, 82
seafood, 94, 158, 239–240. *See also* fish
    allergies to, 174, 175
    in DASH diet, 12, 16
    and heart health, 6, 80
    and hunger, 40
    in Med-DASH plan, 90, 94
    in Mediterranean diet, 4, 6, 10, 12, 16
    protein in, 85
seeds, 92, 103
    allergies to, 175
    antioxidants in, 54
    in DASH diet, 11, 12, 14, 16
    and hunger, 40
    in Med-DASH plan, 90, 92
    in Mediterranean diet, 12
    polyphenols in, 50
serotonin, 46
servings of foods
    on food labels, 154–157
    on jump-start plan, 112–114, 116
    on long-term eating plan, 128–130
Seven Countries Study, 16–17
SFA. *See* saturated fats
smoking, 27, 55
smoothies, 67, 95, 134–135
sodium intake, 154
soy allergy, 174
soy milk, 134
spices. *See* herbs and spices
starches, 78, 85, 98. *See also specific*
    types, e.g.: rice
statins, 28–29, 56
Strong Women Stay Young (Miriam
    Nelson), 229
sugars, 85–86
    absorption of, 95
    in beverages, 86

calories from, 78
carbs breaking down into, 85
and diabetes, 42–43, 58, 59
excessive, 8
in fruits, 86, 94
and gut microbiota, 50, 70
and heart health, 34
and hunger, 40
in Med-DASH diet, 110
and metabolic syndrome, 30
in protein bars, 67
and triglyceride levels, 29
types of, 85
and weight loss, 69

tea, 50, 132
tomatoes, 162
trans fats, 33, 34, 82
traveling, meals when, 171–172
triglycerides
    and belly fat, 40
    and blood sugar surges, 36
    and DASH diet, 15, 19
    and diabetes, 57–58
    and fiber in diet, 98
    from fructose, 86
    and heart disease, 22–24, 28–32, 34
    and high glycemic foods, 42
    and inflammation, 80
    and MUFA-rich fats, 85
    and omega-3 fats, 83
types 1 and 2 diabetes. *See* diabetes/
    type 1 and type 2 diabetes

vegans, 84
vegetables, 94–95
    anti-inflammatory properties of,
        51–52
    antioxidants in, 45, 50, 54, 55, 78

vegetables (*cont.*)
  and blood sugar, 42
  color range of, 101
  in DASH diet, 4, 11, 14
  fiber in, 34, 58, 87, 88
  and hunger, 37, 40, 74
  in juices and smoothies, 67
  in Med-DASH plan, 17, 90,
    94–95
  in Mediterranean diet, 4, 16, 17
  and osteoporosis, 61–62
  phytochemicals in, 78
  polyphenols in, 50
  for spaghetti, 102
vegetarians, 10–11, 14, 47, 84, 95
vitamin A, 46, 78
vitamin C, 54, 94–95
vitamin D, 61, 78, 96
vitamin E, 54, 78
vitamin K, 54, 61–62, 78
vitamins
  antioxidant, 54
  fat-soluble, 78

food sources of, 87, 93, 94, 97,
  103, 160
and Med-DASH plan, 26, 90

waist size, 32, 40, 52–53, 103
water, 124, 132
weight, 37–44. *See also* obesity
  and body-mass index, 38–39
  and calorie intake, 71–72
  and cancer risk, 56
  genetic risk for overweight, 70
  and gut microbiota, 46–47
  health effects of overweight, 70
  and inflammation, 52–53
  and metabolic syndrome, 30–31
  myths about losing, 68–69
  need to lose weight, 70
wine, 4, 29, 50, 55, 133
women, heart disease and, 32–33,
  52–53
work, meals at, 171

yogurt, 133, 154, 166

ABOUT THE AUTHOR

MARLA HELLER, MS, RD, is a registered dietitian, and holds a master of science in human nutrition and dietetics from the University of Illinois at Chicago (UIC), where she also completed doctoral course work in public health, with an emphasis in behavior sciences and health promotion. She is experienced in a wide variety of nutrition counseling specialties and has taught thousands of people how to adopt the DASH diet. She has been an adjunct clinical instructor in the Department of Human Nutrition and Dietetics at UIC, teaching courses on food science and nutrition counseling. At the University of Illinois Medical Center, she was a dietitian working in the Cardiac Step-Down Unit, the Cardiac Intensive Care Unit, and the Heart-Lung Transplant Unit. She was a civilian dietitian with the U.S. Navy and most recently worked for the U.S. Department of Health and Human Services, including the Healthy Weight Collaborative.

In addition to writing the *New York Times* bestsellers *The DASH Diet Action Plan* and *The DASH Diet Weight Loss Solution*, Marla contributed the four-week menu plan for *Win the Weight Game* by Sarah, the Duchess of York. She has been a featured nutrition expert for many national print, television, radio, Internet, and social media platforms. She is a spokesperson for the Greater Midwest

Affiliate of the American Heart Association and a past president of the Illinois Dietetic Association, from which she received their prestigious Emerging Leader Award.

Marla lives with her husband, Richard, and enjoys cooking, gardening, and finding exciting new restaurants.

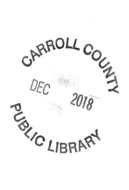